Risk Management in Emergency Medicine

Editors

MICHAEL B. WEINSTOCK
GITA PENSA

EMERGENCY MEDICINE CLINICS OF NORTH AMERICA

www.emed.theclinics.com

Consulting Editor
AMAL MATTU

February 2025 • Volume 43 • Number 1

ELSEVIER

1600 John F. Kennedy Boulevard • Suite 1800 • Philadelphia, Pennsylvania, 19103-2899

http://www.theclinics.com

**EMERGENCY MEDICINE CLINICS OF NORTH AMERICA Volume 43, Number 1
February 2025 ISSN 0733-8627, ISBN-13: 978-0-443-29602-4**

Editor: Joanna Gascoine
Developmental Editor: Varun Gopal

Emergency Medicine Clinics of North America (ISSN 0733-8627) is published quarterly by Elsevier Inc., 360 Park Avenue South, New York, NY, 10010-1710. Months of issue are February, May, August, and November. Business and Editorial Offices: 1600 John F. Kennedy Boulevard, Suite 1800, Philadelphia, PA 19103-2899. Customer Service Office: 6277 Sea Harbor Drive, Orlando, FL 32887-4800. Periodicals postage paid at New York, NY, and additional mailing offices. Subscription prices are $100.00 per year (US students), $396.00 per year (US individuals), $220.00 per year (international students), $515.00 per year (international individuals), $100.00 per year (Canadian students), $472.00 per year (Canadian individuals). For institutional access pricing please contact Customer Service via the contact information below. International air speed delivery is included in all *Clinics*' subscription prices. All prices are subject to change without notice. Orders, claims, and journal inquiries: Please visit our Support Hub page https://service.elsevier.com for assistance.

Reprints. For copies of 100 or more of articles in this publication, please contact the Commercial Reprints Department, Elsevier Inc., 360 Park Avenue South, New York, NY 10010-1710. Tel.: 212-633-3874; Fax: 212-633-3820; E-mail: reprints@elsevier.com.

Emergency Medicine Clinics of North America is covered in *MEDLINE/PubMed (Index Medicus), Current Contents/Clinical Medicine, EMBASE/Excerpta Medica, BIOSIS, SciSearch, CINAHL, ISI/BIOMED*, and *Research Alert.*

Contributors

CONSULTING EDITOR

AMAL MATTU, MD
Professor and Vice Chair of Academic Affairs, Department of Emergency Medicine, University of Maryland School of Medicine, Baltimore, Maryland

EDITORS

MICHAEL B. WEINSTOCK, MD
Emergency Medicine Attending Physician, Adena Health System, Director of Research and Scholarly Activity, Adena Health System GME, Ohio; Professor of Emergency Medicine, Adjunct, The Wexner Medical Center at The Ohio State University, Columbus, Ohio

GITA PENSA, MD
Adjunct Associate Professor, Department of Emergency Medicine, Brown University, Warren Alpert School of Medicine, Providence, Rhode Island

AUTHORS

KIMBERLY BAMBACH, MD
Assistant Professor, Department of Emergency Medicine, The Ohio State University, Columbus, Ohio

FERNANDA CALIENES CERPA, MD, PGY-2
Emergency Medicine Physician, Emergency Department, Carolinas Medical Center, Charlotte, North Carolina

TERRY MARC CALVERT, JD
Attorney at Law, Calvert, Leever & Ostler, Cypress, Texas

ILENE CLAUDIUS, MD
Professor, Department of Emergency Medicine, UCLA, Los Angeles, California; Physician Specialist, Department of Emergency Medicine, Harbor-UCLA Medical Center, Torrance, California

FRANCESCA COCCHIARALE, DO
Resident Physician, PGY-2, Family Medicine, Adena Regional Medical Center, Chillicothe, Ohio

STEPHEN ANTHONY COLUCCIELLO, MD
Vice Chair and Clinical Professor, Emergency Medicine, Carolinas Medical Center, Wake Forest Medical School, Charlotte, North Carolina

MATTHEW DELANEY, MD
Associate Professor, Department of Emergency Medicine, University of Alabama at Birmingham, Birmingham, Alabama

JONATHAN A. EDLOW, MD
Professor, Department of Emergency Medicine, Harvard Medical School; Physician, Emergency Medicine, Beth Israel Deaconess Medical Center, Boston, Massachusetts

MARK GNATOWSKI Jr, JD
Active Member, Ohio Bar, Columbus, Ohio

KELLY WONG HEIDEPRIEM, MD
Clinical Assistant Professor, Department of Family Medicine, University of South Dakota Sanford School of Medicine, Sioux Falls, South Dakota

VERONICA M. HEITSCH, MD, MBOE
Rheumatologist, Vice President of Quality & Safety, GME Medical Director of Quality Improvement, Adena Health System, Ohio

COLIN KAIDE, MD, FACEP, FAAEM
Clinical Professor, Medical Education, Department of Emergency Medicine, The Ohio State University, Columbus, Ohio

ANDREW KENDLE, MD
Staff Physician, Department of Emergency Medicine, University of California at San Francisco Medical Center, San Francisco, California

ALYSSA KETTLER, MD
Fellow, Pediatric Emergency Medicine, Department of Emergency Medicine, Harbor-UCLA Medical Center, Torrance, California

BROCK LANDRUM, MD
Chief Resident, Department of Emergency Medicine, Summa Health System, Akron, Ohio

EVIE G. MARCOLINI, MD, MBE
Associate Professor of Emergency Medicine and Neurology, Emergency Medicine and Neurocritical Care, Dartmouth-Hitchcock Medical Center, Lebanon, New Hampshire

KEVIN MARKOWSKI, MD
Clinical Associate Professor of Emergency Medicine, Northeast Ohio Medical University, Rootstown, Ohio; Regional Quality Director, US Acute Care Solutions, Canton, Ohio; Department of Emergency Medicine, Summa Health System, Akron, Ohio

MICHAEL PALLACI, DO, FACEP, FACOEP
Professor of Emergency Medicine, Northeast Ohio Medical University, Rootstown, Ohio; Clinical Professor of Emergency Medicine, Ohio University Heritage College of Osteopathic Medicine, Athens, Ohio; Director, Summa Health System Simulation Medicine Fellowship Program, Medical Director, Virtual Care Simulation Lab, Core Faculty, Emergency Medicine Residency Program, Department of Emergency Medicine, Summa Health System, Akron, Ohio

GITA PENSA, MD
Adjunct Associate Professor, Department of Emergency Medicine, Brown University, Warren Alpert School of Medicine, Providence, Rhode Island

MARC A. PROBST, MD, MS
Assistant Professor, Director of Adult Research, Department of Emergency Medicine, Columbia University Irving Medical Center, New York, New York

ROBERT RAINER, MD
Resident, Department of Emergency Medicine, The Ohio State University, Columbus, Ohio

CHRISTOPHER E. SAN MIGUEL, MD, MED, FAAEM, FACEP
Associate Professor – Clinical, Department of Emergency Medicine, The Ohio State University College of Medicine, Columbus, Ohio

PATRICK SILER, MD
Associate Professor, Department of Emergency Medicine, University of Alabama at Birmingham, Birmingham, Alabama

NICOLE TYCZYNSKA, MD
Attending Physician, Pennsylvania Hospital and Penn Presbyterian Medical Center; Associate Professor of Emergency Medicine PSOM at University of Pennsylvania, Pennsylvania Hospital, Philadelphia, Pennsylvania

MICHAEL B. WEINSTOCK, MD
Professor of Emergency Medicine, Adjunct, The Wexner Medical Center at The Ohio State University, Columbus, Ohio; Emergency Medicine Attending Physician, Adena Health System, Director of Research and Scholarly Activity, Adena Health System GME, Ohio

REBECCA E. YOUNKER, Esq, JD, PA-C
Associated at Troutman Pepper, Philadelphia, Pennsylvania

Contents

Foreword: Risk Management in Emergency Medicine   xiii

Amal Mattu

Preface: Risk Management in Emergency Medicine   xv

Michael B. Weinstock and Gita Pensa

Medical Malpractice Stress Syndrome   1

Francesca Cocchiarale, Mark Gnatowski Jr., and Gita Pensa

> The majority of physicians will face at least one medical malpractice claim over the course of their careers. The stress caused by medical malpractice claims can lead to litigation stress or malpractice stress syndrome. Physicians experiencing a claim may have strained family relationships, worsening anxiety and depression, and burnout, and have higher rates of medical errors. In such cases, physicians should seek support of their legal counsel and from a licensed professional therapist. Above all, physicians should remember that malpractice claims are an occupational hazard and not a sign that they are a bad physician.

Balancing the Legal Risk to the Clinician with the Medical Interests of the Patient   9

Michael B. Weinstock, Veronica M. Heitsch, and Marc A. Probst

> The balance between risk of missing serious disease and potential harms from over testing involves knowledge of the literature, familiarity of clinical guidelines, incorporation of clinical decision tools where appropriate, use of metacognition to be aware of cognitive decisions to respond and use of shared decision-making in the context of a patient's presentation and with the *guidance* of the clinician.

Medical Malpractice Epidemiology: Adults and Pediatrics   19

Kelly Wong Heidepriem

> For emergency medicine physicians, being named in a malpractice suit is not an *if*, it is a *when*. By the age of 55 years, 68% of emergency physicians have been sued. In the following article, we review the most common factors shared by closed claims in adult and pediatric patients from emergency departments and acute care settings. Our hope is that by identifying shared characteristics, we may improve patient care and reduce litigation risk.

Medicolegally Protective Documentation in Emergency Medicine   29

Michael Pallaci, Kevin Markowski, and Brock Landrum

> More than 75% of emergency physicians will be named in a malpractice suit over the course of their careers. When a case is brought to trial, it is the chart that will be the primary source of information, not the faded

memories of an encounter that happened years in the past. Being mindful of all 3 audiences that the chart is generated for and developing techniques to adequately address all 3 should be the focus of the clinician when documenting a patient encounter.

Pediatric High-Risk Conditions   41

Alyssa Kettler and Ilene Claudius

Meningitis, appendicitis, and testicular torsion are among the most common conditions resulting in malpractice litigation in Pediatric Emergency Medicine. With meningitis, most litigation claims involved patients <2 years old. Notably, 25% of patients had no fever and many lacked classic signs of meningitis. For appendicitis, nearly 3/4 of litigated cases claimed delayed/missed diagnosis. A non-diagnostic ultrasound (eg, no appendix visualized) has a negative predictive value of only 86%. Finally, testicular torsion carries a 34-42% testicular loss rate and 10% of patients with torsion only present with isolated abdominal pain. Atypical presentations must be considered and clear return precautions are imperative.

Chest Pain-Specific Legal Risk   57

Matthew DeLaney and Patrick Siler

Chest pain is a common chief complaint in the emergency department. When looking at patients with chest pain cases of acute coronary syndrome, pulmonary embolism and aortic dissection account for the majority of cases that involve an allegation of malpractice. While it is likely impossible to catch all these cases having a structured approach to these patients may improve outcomes for both patients and clinicians.

Misdiagnosis of Acute Headache: Mitigating Medico-legal Risks   67

Jonathan A. Edlow

Headache is a common complaint of patients in the emergency department. The large majority of them have self-limited causes but some have life, limb, brain, or vision-threatening secondary causes. The job of the emergency physicians is to distinguish the 2 groups. This article focuses on clinical tips to avoid or at least mitigate medico-legal risk in patients with headache. Each process of care—history, physical examination, laboratory testing, brain imaging, spinal fluid analysis, specialist consultation, and documentation—will be considered.

Neurologic Specific Risk: Strokes, Lytics, and Litigation   81

Evie G. Marcolini

Misdiagnosis in Emergency Medicine can be associated with patient harm, with neurologic diagnoses among the most common conditions to confound physicians. These are often complex, time-sensitive and nuanced, offering opportunity for mimics and chameleons to make assessment, diagnosis and treatment challenging. This article discusses the legal considerations pertinent to neurologic diagnoses for the emergency physician, including assessment, diagnosis, treatment, transfer and documentation in order to ensure excellent patient care as well as protection from liability.

Abdominal Pain-Specific Legal Risk   93

Andrew Kendle and Colin Kaide

> Abdominal pain accounts for approximately 10% of emergency depart-
> ment visits and 4% to 6% of litigation. Clinical history and examination
> are important, as all diagnostic testing has limitations. Specific patholo-
> gies, such as appendicitis, warrant a review of factors increasing risk. In
> all cases, documentation of prompt communication with consultants can
> be protective in the event of any unforeseen delays in care. Careful atten-
> tion should be paid to special populations including patients with cancer,
> diabetes, and patients with postsurgical, geriatric, and bariatric surgery.

**Legal Risk to the Emergency Medicine Resident in Training and Attending
Supervisors**   115

Nicole Tyczynska and Rebecca E. Younker

> Medical malpractice is an inevitable truth of being a practicing provider.
> Despite awareness of malpractice risk, education on understanding the le-
> gal landscape and protecting oneself from being named in a malpractice
> claim is sorely underrepresented in medical school and residency curric-
> ula. This review summarizes what is known about the legal risks to the res-
> ident in training and the attending physician supervisor. It also explores the
> legal landscape for physicians practicing and supervising telehealth
> encounters.

Navigating Supervision of Advanced Practice Providers   131

Robert Rainer and Kimberly Bambach

> Current trends demonstrate that the proportion and complexity of emer-
> gency care provided by advanced practice providers (APPs) is increasing,
> which underscores the importance of emergency physician supervision
> and support. Laws governing supervision vary between physician assis-
> tants and nurse practitioners, with the latter legally able to practice inde-
> pendently in some states. Regardless of the supervision model,
> emergency medicine professional organizations advocate for physician-
> led teams. Communication lapses and contradictory documentation with
> errors and omission are potential sources of medical error and risk. Ensur-
> ing appropriate oversight with consideration of the APPs experience and
> documenting appropriately may minimize legal risk.

**Understanding Against Medical Advice, Informed Consent, and Emergency Medical
Treatment and Labor Act**   139

Fernanda Calienes Cerpa and Stephen Anthony Colucciello

> As emergency medicine physicians, we engage in informed consent, have
> conversations with patients leaving against medical advice, and screen
> them daily. Better understanding these concepts and processes can im-
> prove patient care.

Clinical Practice Guidelines and Medical Malpractice Risk   **155**

Christopher E. San Miguel

While clinical practice guidelines (CPGs) were developed to help improve patient care, they have increasingly been used as evidence in medical malpractice lawsuits. They are used by both sides in malpractice litigation as a surrogate for the standard of care. Providing care compliant with a CPG can be protective for physicians, but it does not completely absolve them of liability. Providing noncompliant care does carry an increased risk of litigation, but there are several defenses that have been successfully used to defend physicians. Effective communication and comprehensive documentation help mitigate the risk incurred by not following a CPG.

Reflections from a Medical Malpractice Defense Attorney: Insights on Avoiding Claims and Lawsuits   **163**

Terry Marc Calvert

Good decision-making, solid notes that show care and a reasonable thought process, and skillful interpersonal dealings with patients and loved ones are keys to avoiding claims and lawsuits related to care in the emergency department (ED). This means taking measures to control the brisk assembly line of work in the ED so that important steps such as assessment, testing, treatment, and communication promptly occur without any dilution in quality. It is crucial that the physician in the ED displays excellent bedside manner, including dealing with an increasing challenging patient population and the family and friends who often accompany them.

EMERGENCY MEDICINE CLINICS OF NORTH AMERICA

FORTHCOMING ISSUES

May 2025
Geriatric Emergency Medicine
Brittany Ellis and Christina Shenvi, *Editors*

August 2025
Hematologic and Oncologic Emergencies
Monica K. Wattana and Molly Estes, *Editors*

November 2025
Pediatric Emergencies
Ann Dietrich and Sean M. Fox, *Editors*

RECENT ISSUES

November 2024
Clinical Ultrasound in the Emergency Department
Michael Gottlieb and Alexis Salerno, *Editors*

August 2024
Environmental and Wilderness Medicine
Cheyenne Falat and Stephanie Lareau, *Editors*

May 2024
Infectious Disease Emergencies
Bradley W. Frazee, Michael S. Pulia and Christopher M. Colbert, *Editors*

EMERGENCY MEDICINE
CLINICS OF NORTH AMERICA

Foreword

Risk Management in Emergency Medicine

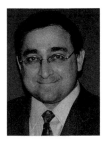

Amal Mattu, MD
Consulting Editor

There's little doubt that emergency medicine is a high-risk specialty. That risk applies to patients as well as clinicians. Patients are at risk by virtue of the conditions with which they present…acute myocardial infarction, stroke, overdose, appendicitis, mesenteric ischemia, compartment syndrome, traumatic injuries…the list can go on and on. Contributing further to that risk is the fact that the health care providers caring for the patients have little information about those patients and need to make decisions quickly, oftentimes without the benefit of the results of tests that have been ordered.

The clinicians themselves are also at risk for all of the reasons listed above, but now add onto that list the fact that the health care system is "challenged," if not broken. Hospital and emergency department overcrowding leads to delays in seeing patients and obtaining test results. Medication shortages abound. Consultants are often not quickly available. The patients themselves are not always able to provide detailed and relevant history, and physical exam findings in certain patients can be unreliable. In recent years, staffing shortages (nurses, patient care techs, and the like) have added to the challenge. Frankly, I am often amazed that more bad outcomes don't occur, given how much the elements seem to conspire against us!

But bad outcomes do occur. Often, they are not preventable. Although we already feel terrible when those bad outcomes occur and we work hard to prevent those bad outcomes from occurring again, that doesn't seem to be enough. The fact is that our society endorses a legal system that sometimes seeks to punish clinicians for bad outcomes whether they were preventable or not.

So, what can we do to decrease the risk of bad outcomes to our patients and to our own practice? I believe that education is the key. We must constantly strive to gain the maximum level of clinical knowledge possible in order to properly diagnose and treat patients. And we must also learn specifically about the common pitfalls that lead to

Emerg Med Clin N Am 43 (2025) xiii–xiv
https://doi.org/10.1016/j.emc.2024.09.001
0733-8627/25/© 2024 Published by Elsevier Inc.

emed.theclinics.com

adverse patient outcomes and that lead to litigation. That latter is what this issue of *Emergency Medicine Clinics of North America* is all about.

In this issue of *Emergency Medicine Clinics of North America*, two experts in emergency medicine risk management, Drs Michael Weinstock and Gita Pensa, have assembled an outstanding group of authors and educators to teach us about how to minimize risk to our patients and ourselves. The group provides us articles that address specific high-risk entities, such as chest pain, abdominal pain, and neurologic disorders, and high-risk patient groups, such as pediatric patients. They also provide articles to teach us about the medical malpractice process to prepare us for that ill-fated day when we ourselves might be subject to litigation. They provide critically important education about supervision of advanced practice providers, and they also discuss the personal stress that defendant physicians face. Finally, they not only bring the teachings of outstanding physicians to us but also bring some advice from attorneys that are involved in medical malpractice litigation.

This issue of *Emergency Medicine of North America* is definitely one of my favorites because it is practical and useful and discusses topics that are not normally taught in training programs or in the textbooks. My hope would be for EVERY emergency clinician to read this issue, cover to cover. It is worth the time. Kudos to the Guest Editors and authors on an excellent contribution to the literature.

Amal Mattu, MD
Department of Emergency Medicine
University of Maryland School of Medicine
Baltimore, MD, USA

E-mail address:
amattu@som.umaryland.edu

Preface

Risk Management in Emergency Medicine

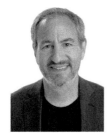
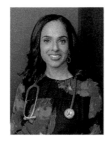

Michael B. Weinstock, MD   Gita Pensa, MD
Editors

It is both curious and understandable that there is such a concern for medical malpractice litigation in emergency medicine: the chance that any average emergency medicine clinician would end up losing in court is very low, but on the other hand, litigation is quite common and there are enormous life implications to simply being named, as you will see in the article on Medical Malpractice Stress Syndrome.

Is there a way to anticipate which patient presentations are prone to rapid deterioration or an inaccurate diagnosis and which patients will then subsequently initiate a lawsuit? Sometimes it is not surprising, but occasionally this can occur out of the blue. Approaching patients with not only a symptoms-based focus (gathering appropriate data with the history and exam) but also a diagnosis-based approach (considering a patient-specific differential and explaining through the documentation why your evaluation and disposition were reasonable) can go a long way toward avoiding the lawsuit being filed in the first place, or toward creating a more powerful defense in the event that a lawsuit is initiated.

Our primary goal, of course, is to improve patient safety, but also to avoid an unnecessary medical-legal odyssey when possible. In an article on patients presenting with headache, we focus on specific high-risk occurrences where we are concerned not only about common entities, such as subarachnoid hemorrhage, but also things more difficult to diagnose, such as idiopathic intracranial hypertension, neck artery dissection, and cerebral venous thrombosis. We focus on abdominal pain, a very common occurrence in the population overall, but a symptom that can occasionally have disastrous consequences. We have a chapter specifically looking at chest pain, still one of the most frequent reasons for litigation.

Emerg Med Clin N Am 43 (2025) xv–xvi
https://doi.org/10.1016/j.emc.2024.05.017
0733-8627/25/© 2024 Published by Elsevier Inc.

emed.theclinics.com

We examine how clinicians collaborate in the emergency department, including physicians working together with nurse practitioners and PAs, faculty overseeing residents, and the consideration of resident liability during training.

How do we balance the long-term health of the patient with the short-term medical-legal concern of the clinician? We do a deep dive into this issue, with specific recommendations on obtaining this sometimes elusive balance in a patient-centric fashion.

We close with real-life experience from a medical malpractice defense attorney with over 30 years of experience. His narrative reflects on ways that specific encounters could have improved patient safety and decreased legal risk by improved bedside interaction with the patient and their family as well as ways of documenting that would have revealed the thought process of the clinician while the patient was still in the emergency department... before an adverse outcome occurred.

This issue of *Emergency Medicine Clinics of North America* is focused on risk management, but we have attempted to go the next level, broadening its scope to explaining risk management not only from the epidemiology but also to a real-world, at the bedside, "in the footsteps" of the emergency medicine clinician approach, to do what we do best: think worst-first, tell a "story" in our note, and provide compassion in healing. We aspire to not only decrease medical-legal exposure but also improve patient safety. In this way, we hope to move from standard of care... to "excellence in care."

Michael B. Weinstock, MD
Adena Health System
Adena Health System GME
Chillicothe, OH, USA

The Wexner Medical Center
The Ohio State University
Columbus, OH, USA

Gita Pensa, MD
Brown University
Warren Alpert School of Medicine
Department of Emergency Medicine
Providence, RI, USA

E-mail addresses:
mweinstock@mweinstock.com (M.B. Weinstock)
gpensa5@gmail.com (G. Pensa)

Medical Malpractice Stress Syndrome

Francesca Cocchiarale, DO[a],*, Mark Gnatowski Jr, JD[b,1],
Gita Pensa, MD[c,2]

KEYWORDS

- Malpractice • Lawsuit • Stress • Litigation • Depression • Anxiety

KEY POINTS

- Most physicians will face at least one medical malpractice claim during their career.
- Litigation stress and medical malpractice stress syndrome can affect many spheres of a clinician's life and can lead to the exacerbation of existing diagnoses including substance abuse disorders, depression, and anxiety.
- Support and self-care are important during litigation to mitigate the impact of litigation stress on a clinician's life.

"YOU HAVE CHILDREN OF YOUR OWN"

A 5 year old boy, Ty,[1] presented to the emergency department (ED) on a Sunday afternoon with a history of abdominal pain, fever, headache, and vomiting for 2 days.[2] Ty was quieter than a typical 5 year old boy, but the parents assured the emergency physician, Dr Charles Chase, that it was common when he was given acetaminophen. Dr Chase attempted to elicit Kernig's sign and Brudzinski's sign, but his findings were equivocal. The parents consented to a lumbar puncture, and Ty's cerebrospinal fluid (CSF) came back with values of 262 red blood cells and 8 white blood cells. Thinking that bacterial meningitis had been ruled out, Dr Chase determined that Ty likely had viral meningitis and sent Ty home with his parents.

By Tuesday, Ty was dead. The CSF culture returned shortly before Dr Chase learned Ty had died: it was *Strep pneumonia* meningitis. Ty's death made the local news, which announced that grief counselors would be made available for his kindergarten classmates. Ty's parents spoke little to the news, broken with grief. All Dr Chase could think

[a] PGY-2, Family Medicine, Adena Regional Medical Center, 4457 State Route 159, Chillicothe, OH 45601, USA; [b] Active Member, Ohio Bar, Columbus, OH, USA; [c] Department of Emergency Medicine, Brown University, Warren Alpert School of Medicine, Providence, RI, USA
[1] Present address: 4457 State Route 159, Chillicothe, OH 45601.
[2] Present address: 145 Meeting Street, Providence, RI 02906.
* Corresponding author.
E-mail address: fcocchiarale@adena.org
Twitter: @GitaPensaMD (G.P.)

Emerg Med Clin N Am 43 (2025) 1–7
https://doi.org/10.1016/j.emc.2024.05.024
emed.theclinics.com
0733-8627/25/© 2024 Elsevier Inc. All rights reserved, including those for text and data mining, AI training, and similar technologies.

was "[s]o much pain, for so many, and it was my doing." He even considered suicide, only being saved by "reasoning that if [he] had already caused so much pain, then [his] suicide would just cause more." A year after Ty's death, he was served with a medical malpractice complaint.

After 2 years of mental anguish, Dr Chase's wife reached a point of exhaustion. She finally broke through to him by saying, "You are stuck on that dead child—you have children of your own to take care of!" He sought counseling and received a post-traumatic stress disorder diagnosis; cognitive therapy and eye movement desensitization response ultimately helped him manage it. So did the end of the case.

Throughout the case, Dr Chase had informed his legal team of his intent to settle. Chase told his counsel, "I could not, would not, give any lawyerly answers on the stand in front of Ty's mom and dad. If asked, I would say I had made a mistake."

Dr Chase settled for $1.1 million. "Ty's parent[s] came over hugging and crying and we finally got to talk. We have talked a lot since."

LITIGATION STRESS AND MEDICAL MALPRACTICE STRESS SYNDROME

The true story described earlier exemplifies the anguish that many physicians feel in the wake of a serious adverse event.[3] We take great pride in providing exemplary medical care to our patients, and when things go wrong, the clinician often also suffers. This in no way negates the suffering of the patients or their family, both perspectives are true and valid. Our focus in this article will be the mental anguish and stress of the physician involved in a case with serious allegations that moves to litigation.

The accusation of malpractice and subsequent prolonged litigation add to the mental distress of the clinician after an adverse outcome. This distress, dubbed litigation stress or medical malpractice stress syndrome (MMSS), is common among physicians who are sued—and unfortunately, many emergency physicians will endure it in their careers. Nearly 75% of emergency physicians in the United States will be named in a malpractice claim.[4]

Litigation stress is a predictable response to this significant long-term stressor. Physicians may have a range of reactions, from annoyance to depression and suicidal ideation. There is no current Diagnostic and Statistical Manual of Mental Disorders-associated diagnosis for litigation stress or malpractice stress syndrome. However, self-reported instances often have cognitive, emotional, physical, spiritual, and interpersonal dimensions. Emotional features include the aforementioned depression, anxiety, isolation, shame, disillusionment shock, overwhelm, and apathy. Cognitively, the physician may struggle to concentrate, have a low tolerance for frustration, and experience difficulty making decisions. Physical symptoms may include those we might recognize in patients under severe stress, such as insomnia, palpitations, gastrointestinal upset, headaches, and shakiness. Spiritually, the physician may withdraw from their spiritual community and lose their sense of purpose or their faith. The physician may also withdraw from, or have conflict within, their interpersonal relationships (**Box 1**).

Box 1	
Impacts of medical malpractice stress syndrome	
Cognitive	Struggle to concentrate, low tolerance for frustration, and difficulty making decisions
Emotional	Depression, anxiety, isolation, shame, and disillusionment
Spiritual	Withdrawal from spiritual community, loss of sense of purpose, loss of faith
Interpersonal	Withdrawal and conflict within personal relationships

Litigation stress and MMSS exist on a continuum, with MMSS having more significant symptoms. The physician with MMSS may experience worsening depression, anxiety, or stress-related physical symptoms. They may have significant difficulties surrounding performance at work and may also have higher rates of medical errors, experience burnout, productivity changes, or have interpersonal issues with co-workers. The physician may also cope by engaging in substance use or may relapse into a substance-use disorder. Family relationships are frequently disrupted. Though physicians are already experiencing an increased risk of suicidality relative to the general population, there is some evidence that suicidality is increased among physicians subject to litigation.[5]

Though all physicians are at risk for malpractice stress syndrome, certain factors may increase the risk. A previous underlying depression or anxiety disorder increases this risk, as does previous substance-use disorder.[6] Cases with more serious outcomes (eg, neurologic devastation, death) or cases in which the defendants feel they made a serious error also increase the risk. Finally, the defendant being subject to high-profile press involvement from the case may also contribute to an increased likelihood. These factors interplay with the extended timeline for litigation, in which each phase has unique stressors. Such phases include initial service of the complaint, deposition (questioning under oath before trial, which requires extensive preparation), trial and any testimony given at trial, and receiving the verdict.

GAINING PERSPECTIVE

A 51 year old male physician presented to the ED with chest pain and dyspnea. A social history uncovered that the man had recently been served with a $10 million medical malpractice complaint. Further questioning revealed severe anxiety and suicidal ideation for the previous 5 days. His cardiac evaluation was negative, and after being seen by a psychiatrist, he received another diagnosis: MMSS.

Litigation can feel like an assault on a physician's identity; leaving one questioning the sacrifices made to become a physician. A physician might find it uncomfortable to see a patient with similar complaints to the one who is suing him, or to perform a procedure associated with the complaint. Posttraumatic symptoms, including flashbacks, rumination, and panic physiology, are common, especially when placed in a situation similar to the adverse event. Sometimes these symptoms can be so severe that they impede a physician's ability to practice and eventually lead to career abandonment. Fear of going to work can create career dissatisfaction and contribute to burnout in an atmosphere that is already quite difficult for emergency physicians.

Although many physicians feel shame when they are sued, litigation is not a sign that one is a poor physician. Of 6779 closed claims in one study, 65.9% were dropped, withdrawn, or dismissed; another 22.8% of claims settled for an average indemnity of $297,709.[7] Of the 515 (7.6%) cases that went to trial, juries returned verdicts for the defendant in 92.6% of cases (477 out of 515). The remaining 7.4% of cases (38 out of 515) were jury verdicts for the plaintiff. Claims reporting major permanent injury had the highest paid-to-closed ratio, and those reporting grave injury had the highest average indemnity of $686,239. Similarly, a case ending in settlement payment may create feelings of anger or shame for the physician, but many lawsuits are settled despite defensible care on the part of the physician. Numerous considerations may go into any decision to settle a case, including the how the overall optics of a case might appear to a jury of laypeople, and the decision to settle may not be in the hands of the physician, depending on their malpractice insurance policy.

Plaintiffs' attorneys may try to make the physician feel like a bad person and a bad physician. This is a deliberate strategy, as skilled plaintiff's attorneys understand the psychology of the physician, and their goal is to obtain the best settlement or verdict possible for their client using whatever legal means they have at their disposal. The physician should take care not to internalize that messaging and instead recognize it as tactical. It is more helpful to consider litigation to be an occupational hazard, as frequent as it is.

STRATEGIES FOR LITIGATION STRESS SUPPORT

"Don't talk about it" is a common admonition to a defendant, despite it being both misguided and unhealthy.[8] Specific events within a case (presentation, documentation, testing, and management) are distinct from the emotional toll borne by the physician. Peer support, therapy, coaching, talking with trusted friends, family, and colleagues can be therapeutic and a healthy way to process the trauma associated with adverse events and litigation.

Working with peer supporters, professional mental health clinicians, or coaches may help the physician put these fears in better perspective and regain confidence in their abilities; in fact Kiser and colleagues performed a trial of 138 physicians randomized to 6 coaching sessions or a control group finding a control group finding that peer coaching is effective at reducing burnout and increasing well-being.[9]

To mitigate litigation stress, physicians must pay attention to their wellness and engage in self-care. Three core pillars can help the physician maintain some stability: exercise, good nutrition, and adequate sleep. The physician must also nurture their personal relationships and schedule time off for nonwork-related and enjoyable activities.

One should consider a reduction in hours or a leave of absence if work becomes a significant stressor or if you experience constant feelings of overwhelm. The physician should try to become educated about the legal process and timeline to gain a better understanding and regain a sense of control. Consider listening to podcasts about litigation, consulting professional society resources, and attending lectures on the topic to become a more confident defendant. However, the physician should not become consumed or ruminate over the litigation. Blocking out time to prepare or learn about litigation may help avoid engaging in catastrophizing and rumination.

Openly discussing litigation within medical culture can help lessen the shame and stigma associated with what has become commonplace. Historically, teaching learners about litigation beyond basic risk management principles and the "anatomy of a lawsuit" lecture has been very rare. This deprives young physicians of any role models of physicians who perform well in litigation or who have incorporated it into who they are as a doctor. Being more open about litigation and how to perform as a defendant with integrity and strategy will eventually help change the shame and terror of the newly named defendant.

Though seeking out support from trusted friends, family, and peers is encouraged, you should only discuss the details of your case and your medical care with your legal team, to avoid waiving attorney–client privilege or client confidentiality. However, the existence of the lawsuit itself and what is in the legal complaint are matters of public record, and therefore not considered "case details." Discussing the fact that litigation is underway and your feelings about the case itself can help you process these difficult emotions.

Consider learning coping and resilience strategies from a licensed professional therapist (eg, cognitive behavioral therapy techniques or acceptance commitment therapy techniques). Knowledge gaps about litigation itself can lead to anticipatory anxiety; books, professional society resources, and other educational materials can help you better understand what to expect during litigation, and how to perform well as a defendant. Learning how to be a meaningful member of the defense team can give physicians an understanding of what they can control, as well as potentially positively influencing the outcome of their case. Catastrophizing is more likely to occur in the absence of real understanding.

Finally, physicians must learn to recognize red flags in themselves that should prompt immediate professional intervention or a leave of absence from work including

- Thoughts of suicide,
- Increased errors or near-misses at work,
- Elevated use of alcohol or other drugs,
- Withdrawal or isolation, and
- Aggression or rage.

Recognizing these as symptoms of MMSS, and not a personal failing of the physician, is an important perspective to encourage. Medical colleagues should also understand the gravity of litigation stress in peers and reach out to physicians that they feel may be struggling under the weight of litigation. Formal peer support programs or informal offerings of assistance can help the clinician feel less alone and confirm that they remain a valued member of their department, regardless of the legal events.

SUMMARY

While we wait for such cultural changes, here we summarize options for a defendant to consider to attend to their own well-being.

A. Wellness and self-care
- Reframe litigation as a difficult event that gives you permission to make changes to support your well-being.
- Attend to exercise, nutrition, and sleep.
- Nurture personal relationships (eg, through quality time).
- Schedule time off from work to do something not associated with work.
- Consider reducing hours or taking a leave of absence if work is a significant stressor or if work produces feelings of overwhelm.
- Be vigilant when using alcohol, other drugs, or sleep aids.
- Do not allow rumination about the litigation consume your waking hours. Schedule time to think, worry, and learn about the process. Use positive distractions to prevent rumination and catastrophizing.
B. Developing your litigation skill set
- Read about malpractice litigation and being a defendant.
- Follow the advice of your legal counsel.
- Consult resources from your professional society.
- Attend lectures and listen to podcasts.
- Know that your preparation will help you become more confident, effective, and less anxious.
C. Investigate support resources
- Sara Charles Physician Litigation Stress Resource Center
- American College of Emergency Physicians List of Resources
- Consult professional society resources
- Seek out peer support, therapy, or coaching

- Speaking with physicians who have previously been sued
- Learn about research-based coping and resilience strategies such as
  - Cognitive behavioral therapy techniques
  - Acceptance commitment therapy techniques
  - Work with a therapist or coach to implement these
- Professional intervention is recommended for physicians with severe symptoms of malpractice stress syndrome

D. Reframe how you think about the litigation process.
- Litigation is an occupational hazard.
- Plaintiff's attorney will attempt to make you feel like a bad person and physician. Do not internalize it.
- Seek support from family and friends.
- Consider joining your institution's peer-support network (if one exists).

CLINICS CARE POINTS

- The average physician in the United States will spend 50.7 months, or 11% of a 40 year career, with at least one open, unresolved malpractice claim.
- Strict adherence to applicable guidelines (eg, from Joint Commission on Accreditation of Healthcare Organizations or Centers for Medicare & Medicaid Services) is a proxy to show that the physician followed the appropriate standard of care.
- Physicians without malpractice claims are more likely to have longer visits, solicit patient opinions, invite further comment, use orientation statements to convey the flow of the visit, and use more humor.
- Among physicians in low-risk specialties, 36% were projected to face their first claim by the age of 45 years, as compared with 88% of physicians in high-risk specialties. By the age of 65 years, 75% of physicians in low-risk specialties and 99% of those in high-risk specialties were projected to face a claim.
- Litigation stress is a common reaction to a malpractice lawsuit, as it may represent a threat to identity of the clinician, and many clinicians report inadequate training or instruction on what to expect during litigation.

DISCLOSURE

The authors have nothing to disclose.

REFERENCES

1. All persons named in this story have had their names changed.
2. Weinstock MB, Klauer KM, Joseph MM, et al. Bouncebacks! Pediatrics. Columbus (OH): Anadem Publishing; 2015. p. 135–66. Case 10: 5-Year-Old Boy with Headache.
3. Pensa G. Medical malpractice stress syndrome. In: Mattu A, Swadron S, editors. CorePendium. Burbank (CA): CorePendium, LLC; 2023. Available at: https://www.emrap.org/corependium/chapter/recUDAOuZUT4od64Y/Medical-Malpractice-Stress-Syndrome. [Accessed 20 January 2024].
4. Jena AB, Seabury S, Lakdawalla D, et al. Malpractice risk according to physician specialty. N Engl J Med 2011;365(7):629–36.
5. Ji YD, Robertson FC, Patel NA, et al. Assessment of Risk Factors for Suicide Among US Health Care Professionals. JAMA Surg 2020;155(8):713–21. https://doi.org/10.1001/jamasurg.2020.1338.

6. Gold KJ, Sen A, Schwenk TL. Details on suicide among US physicians: data from the National Violent Death Reporting System. Gen Hosp Psychiatr 2013;35(1): 45–9. https://doi.org/10.1016/j.genhosppsych.2012.08.005.
7. Wong KE, Parikh PD, Miller KC, et al. Emergency Department and Urgent Care Medical Malpractice Claims 2001-15. West J Emerg Med 2021 Feb 15;22(2): 333–8. PMID: 33856320; PMCID: PMC7972370.
8. Much of what follows stems from the experience of one of the authors.
9. Kiser SB, Sterns JD, Lai PY, et al. Physician coaching by professionally trained peers for burnout and well-being: a randomized clinical trial. JAMA Netw Open 2024;7(4):e245645.

Balancing the Legal Risk to the Clinician with the Medical Interests of the Patient

Michael B. Weinstock, MD[a,b,c,]*, Veronica M. Heitsch, MD[a],
Marc A. Probst, MD, MS[d]

KEYWORDS

- Emergency medicine • Risk management • Balance risk and benefit

KEY POINTS

- There is significant and understandable practice variation in emergency medicine (EM).
- When considering evaluation and management of patients, the clinician should be aware that their own level of risk aversion may be different than that of their patients.
- Despite these inherent aspects of the practice of medicine (prone to the human condition of both the patient and the clinician), optimal care of patients may be achieved by knowledge of the literature, use of clinical guidelines and clinical decision instruments, understanding how metacognition can mitigate our own cognitive biases, and the use of shared decision-making to guide clinical management.

THE SCENARIO

A 19-year-old woman with no significant past medical history presents to the emergency department (ED) with 2 days of constant, squeezing chest pain, which is pleuritic in nature. There is no radiation or diaphoresis. She also reports blood-streaked sputum. She has a temperature of 101.2°F and has been exposed to 2 siblings who have similar respiratory symptoms. She is currently taking oral contraceptives and is a nonsmoker. Her vital signs are normal including a room air oxygen saturation of 97%. She has no subjective or objective pain or swelling of the lower extremities.

[a] Adena Health System, 272 Hospital Road, Chillicothe, OH 45601, USA; [b] Adena Health System GME, OH, USA; [c] The Wexner Medical Center at the Ohio State University, 410 West 10th Avenue, Columbus, OH 43210, USA; [d] Department of Emergency Medicine, Columbia University Irving Medical Center, New York, NY, USA
* Corresponding author.
E-mail address: mweinstock@mweinstock.com
Twitter: @embouncebacks (M.B.W.); @probstMD (M.A.P.)

Emerg Med Clin N Am 43 (2025) 9–18
https://doi.org/10.1016/j.emc.2024.05.021
emed.theclinics.com
0733-8627/25/© 2024 Elsevier Inc. All rights reserved, including those for text and data mining, AI training, and similar technologies.

THE CHOICES:

- *Order laboratory testing including a D-dimer to rule-out pulmonary embolism (PE)*
- *Order a chest computed tomography angiogram to rule out PE*
- *Order a chest radiograph to assess for pneumonia*
- *Reassure the patient that she has an acute viral infection and does not need further testing*
- *Use shared decision-making (SDM) to guide testing with the understanding that PE is very unlikely, but that objective testing in the ED is medically reasonable*

There is not one correct answer, as all of these choices seem reasonable. It is interesting that patients with an identical complaint can be managed so differently. We will explore the delicate balance between best patient care with the unspoken considerations inherent to the practice of emergency medicine- that the clinician's care may be influenced by defensive medicine, fear of legal action, and the volume and acuity of other patients in the ED, all in an attempt to balance the 3 S's of emergency medicine: safety, speed, and satisfaction.

PRACTICE VARIATION

At the margins, the practice of emergency medicine is largely uniform; a patient with typical symptoms of a myocardial infarction and an electrocardiogram (ECG) with ST-segment elevations will go emergently to the catheterization laboratory. Similarly, a patient with an ankle sprain and normal radiographs will be discharged with a splint. When the level of uncertainty is higher, there is an existential question that arises: How do we balance the best medical interests of the patient with the legal risk to the clinician?[1]

There is a reason that our trade is called the "practice" or "art" of medicine; we are different than airline pilots who use firm protocols based on objective information shown on instruments while operating a machine created by humans. Our "art" is subject to our ability to obtain data from patients who may be ill, intoxicated, altered, demented, unwilling to give an accurate history, or preverbal. Patients may have a different understanding of terms that clinicians take for granted, for example, "shortness of breath."[2] There are many reasons why clear and effective communication can be compromised in the ED setting. Additionally, we often do not obtain appropriate data on which to base a decision, and attempts to guess patient expectations are not always correct.[3] Finally, even when evaluating similar patients, there remains a significant amount of practice variation[4,5] as well as inaccurate risk estimates sometimes disproportionally accounting for "typical" symptoms and risk factors.[6]

Considering the above patient scenario, many factors might factor into the decision to pursue further objective testing versus providing simple verbal reassurance. These factors may include the patient or family's concerns and expectations, the clinician's last worst case (ie, recency bias), the flow of the department, availability and timeliness of resources, as well as the patient and physician's understanding and tolerance of risk, which could certainly be prone to error.[7]

It is easy to see how this presentation would be managed differently by various clinicians.

METRICS: APPROPRIATE OR AN IMPEDIMENT TO SAFE CARE?

Apart from the well-known medico-legal risks that all emergency physicians (EPs) face in the United States, there are other external factors that influence medical decision-making, including a desire to meet patients' expectations and to meet departmental or institutional metrics. Fenton and colleagues found that patients in the highest patient satisfaction quartile had higher health care expenditures and a higher mortality.[8] Could it be that changing our normal "best practice" to meet the perception of a patient's expectations leads to *worse* care and outcomes? Ong and colleagues studied 272 patients with upper respiratory infections in 10 academic EDs finding that physicians were more likely to prescribe antibiotics when they thought patients expected them, but they were only able to correctly predict those expectations 27% of the time.[9]

There are a range of metrics, but not all are equivalent; for example, for ED patients with chest pain, a major adverse cardiac event (MACE) is defined by the original HEART (History, ECG, Age, Risk factors, Troponin) validation study as death, myocardial infarction (MI) or revascularization at 6 weeks,[10] whereas the HEART pathway (with serial troponin assays) defines MACE as death or MI at 30 days.[11] It is curious that these outcome measures are grouped together, as they are not equivalent. Take, for example, an appropriately diagnosed patient with chest pain who is discharged home from the ED and undergoes revascularization 2 weeks post-ED visit. This patient would still count as a MACE, the same as a death or MI, while the ED care may have been completely appropriate and met all quality metrics.[12]

Half of ED clinicians are comfortable with a miss rate of only 1 out of 1000 to 1 out of 10,000[13,14]; however, the American College of Emergency Physicians (ACEP) states in a 2018 Clinical Policy on Acute Coronary Syndromes (ACS) that (1) there are limitations in diagnostic technology, (2) there is harm associated with false-positive test results, and (3) "the majority of patients and providers would agree that a missed diagnosis rate of 1% to 2% for 30-day MACE in Non-ST-Elevation ACS is acceptable."[15] (Note that the 2 cited survey studies were conducted before the 2018 ACEP Clinical Policy.) This is the essence of our discussion; sometimes fear of litigation or simply fear of misdiagnosis drives evaluation (testing) and management (admission and medications) to the point that now "the risk of the test is *greater than* the risk of missing the disease."

RISK TO THE PATIENT

When do we decide to order a test (or an intervention such as admission)? The theoretic answer is when the risk of the test is *less than* the risk of missing the disease. Though there are some other subtleties, it is easy to see how a clinician who has recently been subject of a legal action or adverse event discussed in peer review or root cause analysis could change their typical practice patterns by ordering tests more frequently. As further studies are published validating clinical decision rules, we find the "acceptable miss rate" with many evaluations approaches 1% to 2%. Attempts to get the sensitivity below that number has the potential to tip the balance to cause harm by overtesting.

- The PE rule out criteria (PERC) rule estimates that in the low-risk group, patients with a negative PERC score will have a 1.4% prevalence of PE.[16]
- As previously described, ACEP defines an acceptable miss rate for non ST-elevation myocardial infarction (nSTEMI) MACE of 1% to 2%[15]
- The Pediatric Emergency Care Applied research Network (PECARN) criteria for pediatric head injury approaches 100% sensitivity for a "clinically important traumatic brain injury (ciTBI)," a level so low that it is thought to be lower that the risk of CT-induced malignancies.[17,18]

Though there is often a risk to the test itself (eg, ionizing radiation from CT scans or coronary artery perforation from a diagnostic catheterization), there are also risks of false-positive findings, sometimes leading to additional testing, which may not improve outcomes[19] while increasing patient anxiety.

The number of *deaths due to preventable harm* is staggering, estimated at over 200,000 per year according to James and colleagues, with "serious harm" being 10 to 20 times as common as lethal harm.[20] Not only is there is a risk to testing but also a risk to admitting patients to the hospital (including falls, nosocomial infections, deep vein thrombosis/PE, and false-positive tests in addition to the expense and hassle of missing work or time away from home).

RISK TO THE CLINICIAN: DEFENSIVE MEDICINE AND LEGAL CONSIDERATIONS

Compounding practice variation is the "elephant in the room": a high prevalence of defensive medicine and concern of potential legal implications for a misdiagnosis or adverse outcome.

Defensive Medicine

Defensive medicine, which may be defined as a deviation from standard medical practice induced by a threat of liability, falls into 2 main categories:

- Assurance behavior (positive defensive medicine): Supplying additional services of marginal or no medical value with the goal to reduce adverse outcomes, deter patients from filing malpractice claims, provide documented evidence of standard of care to pre-empt future legal action, or higher scores on patient satisfaction surveys.
- Avoidance behavior (negative defensive medicine): Where clinicians distance themselves from sources of legal risk by refusing certain procedures or patients.

On balance, defensive medicine is thought to lead to an additional 5% to 13% in health care costs with some estimates of yearly costs approximating hundreds of billions of dollars to the US health care system.[21–24] Studdert and colleagues surveyed 824 physicians in 4 high-risk specialties, including EM, obstetrics, radiology, and surgery, and found that 93% of respondents admitted to practicing defensive medicine, specifically[25]:

- Ordering unnecessary CT, MRI, or radiographs: 76%
- Unnecessarily referring patients to specialists: 52%
- Often prescribing more medicine than medically indicated: 30%
- Admitting patients to the hospital: 19%
- Obtaining a cardiac workup: 15%

Kanzaria and colleagues surveyed a national sample of 478 EPs and found 97% reported at least some of the advanced imaging studies they personally ordered were medically unnecessary.[26] The main perceived factors were fear of missing a low-probability diagnosis and fear of litigation.

These authors recommend avoiding practicing *defensive* medicine, but to evaluate and document in a way that is *defensible*.

Legal Considerations

Most EPs will be named in a lawsuit at some point during their career. By age of 55 years, up to 75% in low-risk specialties and up to 99% in high-risk specialties will be named in a medical legal action.[27] The average physician spends over 4 years of their career (11% of a 40 year career) in an unresolved, open malpractice claim,[28] so it is not surprising that physicians would be concerned with the potential legal implications of their medical decisions.

The good news for physicians is that over 70% of suits are dismissed, as detailed by Carlson and colleagues who evaluated almost 9.5 million visits to the ED.[29] Wong and colleagues reviewed 6779 closed claims between 2001 and 2015 finding that 66% were dropped, withdrawn, or dismissed and that only 7.6% went to trial, but of those, 92.6% had jury verdicts for the defendant.[30]

Did a lawsuit change practice patterns? Carlson and colleagues evaluated 65 physicians named in a medical malpractice action and compared them to 140 matched controls, finding that there was not a change in measures of care intensity or speed, but there was an increase in patient satisfaction scores.[31]

HOW DO WE OBTAIN THE "BALANCE"?

So how do we obtain the balance of excellence in care of our patients with our own concern for negative implication of our actions, such as a patient complaint, poor patient satisfaction scores, evaluation in peer review, or legal action?

WE PROPOSE 5 SPECIFIC ACTIONS

1. Knowledge of the literature
2. Using guidelines to support practice patterns
3. Use of clinical decision instruments, within the context of each individual patient's presentation
4. Understanding of cognitive biases that may lead us astray (ie, cognitive decisions to respond [CDRs] as described by Pat Croskerry)[32–34]
5. Use of SDM with the *guidance* of the emergency clinician

SPECIFIC ACTIONS

1. Knowledge of the literature

   Understanding the literature helps streamline the approach to diagnosis and potentially avoids false-positive tests that may result in delays of diagnosis/disposition, inappropriate therapies, or further testing. There are many ways EPs can continue to expand their knowledge of the literature, including regular reading of EM journals, subscriptions to evidenced-based email summaries, listening to high-quality continuing medical education audio products, and attending yearly EM conferences. Using the example of patients presenting with possible ACS, knowledge of the risk-stratification literature could lead ED clinicians to discharging appropriate patients more frequently.

   - A systematic review and meta-analysis of North American patients with chest pain revealed that only 0.7% of low-risk HEART score patients had a MACE within 30 days to 6 weeks.[35] This lends further support for an outpatient evaluation and disposition decisions for patients in North American with a low-risk HEART score.
   - In patients with 2 negative troponin tests, an interpretable and nonischemic ECG, and nonconcerning vital signs, the risk of a clinically relevant adverse cardiac event is extremely low,[36,37] further confirming outpatient evaluation of patients with chest pain after a negative ED evaluation.
   - Among patients who do have a non-STEMI (not simply a negative ED evaluation), the 6 month risk for a sudden cardiac death was only 0.79%.[38]

2. Using clinical practice guidelines to support practice patterns

   Knowledge of accepted clinical guidelines from respected sources, especially from EM professional groups such as The Americal College of Emergency

Physicians (ACEP) and The Society for Academic Emergency Medicine (SAEM), can help to streamline and expedite diagnostic testing and disposition decisions.

- As previously detailed, the ACEP on ACS defines an "acceptable miss rate" for MACE of 1% to 2%.[15]
- The 2019 ACEP guidelines on acute nontraumatic headache give a level B recommendation that in patients with a normal neurologic examination, a negative noncontrast CT performed within 6 hours of symptom onset can be performed to rule out nontraumatic subarachnoid hemorrhage.[39]
- The 2021 Guidelines for Reasonable and Appropriate Care (GRACE) guidelines on recurrent, low-risk chest pain in the ED recommend minimal testing for those with a recent provocative cardiac evaluations.[40]

3. Use of clinical decision instruments, within the context of each individual patient's presentation
- The 2019 ACEP headache guidelines mentioned earlier recommend using the Ottawa SAH rule[41] as it has high sensitivity to exclude SAH.[41]
- The PECARN clinical decision rule states that in patients aged under 2 years with a normal Glasgow Coma Scale, without palpable skull fracture, without a severe mechanism or loss of consciousness of 5 seconds or longer, and without altered mental status, the presence of a "ciTBI" is exceedingly low (<0.02%) and that the use of brain imaging is more likely to cause a CT-induced malignancy than to help the patient.[17]
- With a concerned parent who requests a CT scan, the earlier examples serve to demonstrate how care can minimize risks of testing while expediting throughput.

4. Understanding cognitive biases that may lead us astray, that is, CDRs as described by Pat Croskerry[32–34]
- Anchoring bias occurs when the clinician "anchors" onto a diagnosis too early in the diagnostic process and does not incorporate subsequently obtained superior data into the decision-making process.
- Diagnosis momentum occurs when a previous diagnosis becomes established and different or new diagnostic considerations are not entertained.
- Triage cuing is when more or less serious diagnoses are prioritized based on an assigned triage level.
- Meta cognition is described as the highest level of decision-making, where we monitor our own thought-making processes to understand where we may be prone to error, and then can utilize "cognitive debiasing."
- Awareness of these biases innate in all of us may serve to help tip the "balance" toward the best health of the patient.

5. Use of SDM with the *guidance* of the emergency clinician[42,43]
- SDM is defined as "a collaborative process in which patients and providers make health care decisions together, taking into account the best evidence available, as well as the patient's values and preferences."[44] SDM allows the clinicians to harness the intuition of the patient and take into account their individual risk tolerance. By eliciting the patient's values and preferences, it can lead to patient-centered care.
- Evidence from a 2019 experimental survey study of potential ED patients suggests that SDM can reduce medico-legal risk for EPs. A national survey of 737 EPs found roughly two-thirds of participants felt that using and documenting SDM would decrease their medico-legal risk.[42,45]

- SDM should occur with the *guidance* of the clinician, not simply to abdicate responsibility for decision-making onto the patient and attempt to avoid responsibility in the event of an adverse outcome.

BRINGING IT ALL HOME

The case vignette described at the beginning of this article presents the ED clinician with a clinical dilemma. The implications for a missed PE could be severe, while subjecting this young female patient to low-yield testing can also be harmful. This scenario highlights how the ED evaluation could be approached very differently by experienced emergency clinicians as well as how the patient's concerns and risk tolerance may factor into the clinical decision-making. There are various reasonable approaches to this clinical scenario with the understanding that the risk of a PE, while being very low, is not zero. Note that the pulmonary embolism rule-out criteria rule cannot be used as the patient is using hormonal therapy (oral contraceptives).[16,46]

Consider these 2 approaches to the patient's presentation, based on further insight into the patient's considerations:

1. With the clinician's explanation that a PE is very unlikely and the presence of an alternative diagnosis (blood-streaked sputum from a vigorous cough due to the presence of acute viral bronchitis), the patient displays understanding the PE could still be present but is *very* unlikely and she decides, through the application of SDM with the *guidance* of the clinician, that she will forgo any diagnostic testing in the ED (such as D-dimer or CT pulmonary angiogram) and return if symptoms progress, worsen, or do not resolve.
2. With the clinician's same explanation, the patient remains concerned as her best friend died of PE exactly 1 year ago. She states that if she is discharged without a definitive diagnosis, she will be emotionally adversely impacted and requests to have diagnostic testing performed in the ED.

Both of these scenarios are *patient centric* and would be viewed as reasonable, provided there was a medical decision-making note detailing the clinicians thought process. An example could read:

Based on the patient's presenting history and exam including normal vital signs, the most likely diagnosis is acute viral bronchitis with chest pain due to pleurisy or a musculoskeletal etiology and the blood-streaked sputum due to a tracheal irritation from forceful coughing. The possibility of PE was considered but thought to be extremely unlikely. This consideration was discussed with the patient and through the process of SDM the reasonable medical options were discussed. After consideration, we agreed that further diagnostic testing such as CT of the chest will be deferred. She understands that PE has not been 100% excluded and agrees to return with increased pain, more hemoptysis, dyspnea, or pain/swelling of the lower extremities. She will follow up with primary care within 2-3 days.

TAKE HOME POINTS

- There is significant and understandable practice variation in emergency medicine.
- When considering evaluation and management of patients, the clinician should be aware that their own level of risk aversion may be different than that of their patients.

- Despite these inherent aspects of the practice of medicine (prone to the human condition of both the patient and the clinician), best care of patients may be achieved by knowledge of the literature, use of clinical guidelines and clinical decision instruments, understanding how metacognition can mitigate our own cognitive biases, and the use of shared decision-making to guide clinical management.

CLINICS CARE POINTS

- Knowledge of the literature will allow for best care and avoidance of extraneous testing and medication.
- Use guidelines to support practice patterns.
- Use clinical decision rules, within the context of each individual patient's presentation.
- Understanding cognitive biases (ie, CDRs as described by Pat Croskerry) will inform the clinician when their thought-making might be prone to error.
- Use SDM with the *guidance* of the emergency clinician.

DISCLOSURE

The authors have nothing to disclose.

REFERENCES

1. Weinstock MB, Mattu A, Hess EP. How do we balance the long-term health of a patient with the short-term risk to the physician? J Emerg Med 2017;53(4):583–5.
2. Mulrow C, Lucey C, Farnett L. Discriminating causes of dyspnea through the clinical examination. J Gen Intern Med 1993;8:383–92.
3. Ohle R, Mc Isaac S, Perry JJ. A simple intervention to reduce your chance of missing an acute aortic dissection. CJEM 2019;21(5):618–21.
4. Sakhnini A, Bisharat N. Practice behavior of emergency department physicians caring for patients with chest pain. Am J Emerg Med 2019;37(6):1210–2.
5. Pines JM, Isserman JA, Szyld D, et al. The effect of physician risk tolerance and the presence of an observation unit on decision making for ED patients with chest pain. Am J Emerg Med 2010;28(7):771–9.
6. Greenslade JH, Sieben N, Parsonage WA, et al. Factors influencing physician risk estimates for acute cardiac events in emergency patients with suspected acute coronary syndrome. Emerg Med J 2020;37(1):2–7. Epub 2019 Nov 12. PMID: 31719104.
7. Rothberg MB, Sivalingam SK, Ashraf J, et al. Patients' and cardiologists' perceptions of the benefits of percutaneous coronary intervention for stable coronary disease. Ann Intern Med 2010;153(5):307–13.
8. Fenton JJ, Jerant AF, Bertakis KD, et al. The cost of satisfaction: a national study of patient satisfaction, health care utilization, expenditures, and mortality. Arch Intern Med 2012;172(5):405–11.
9. Ong S, Nakase J, Moran GJ, et al. Antibiotic use for emergency department patients with upper respiratory infections: prescribing practices, patient expectations, and patient satisfaction. Ann Emerg Med 2007;50(3):213–20.

10. Backus BE, Six AJ, Kelder JC, et al. A prospective validation of the HEART score for chest pain patients at the emergency department. Int J Cardiol 2013;168(3): 2153–8.
11. Mahler SA, Lenoir KM, Wells BJ, et al. Safely identifying emergency department patients with acute chest pain for early discharge. Circulation 2018;138(22):2456–68.
12. Weinstock MB, Finnerty NM, Pallaci M. Time to move on: redefining chest pain outcomes. J Am Heart Assoc 2019;8(12):e012542.
13. Than MP, Herbert M, Flaws D, et al. What is an acceptable risk of major adverse cardiac event in chest pain patients soon after discharge from the Emergency Department? A clinical survey. Int J Cardiol 2013;166(3):752–4.
14. Weinstock MD, Pallaci M, Mattu A, et al. Most clinicians are still not comfortable sending chest pain patients home with a very low risk of 30-day major adverse cardiac event (MACE). J Urgent Care Med 2021;15(5):17–21.
15. Tomaszewski CA, Nestler D, Shah KH, et al. American College of Emergency Physicians Clinical Policies Subcommittee on Suspected Non-ST-Elevation Acute Coronary Syndromes. Clinical policy: critical issues in the evaluation and management of emergency department patients with suspected non-ST-elevation acute coronary syndromes. Ann Emerg Med 2018;72:e65–106.
16. Kline JA, Mitchell AM, Kabrhel C, et al. Clinical criteria to prevent unnecessary diagnostic testing in emergency department patients with suspected pulmonary embolism. J Thromb Haemostasis 2004;2(8):1247–55.
17. Kuppermann N, Holmes JF, Dayan PS, et al. Identification of children at very low risk of clinically-important brain injuries after head trauma: a prospective cohort study [published correction appears in Lancet. 2014 Jan 25;383(9914):308]. Lancet 2009;374(9696):1160–70.
18. Schonfeld D, Bressan S, Da Dalt L, et al. Pediatric Emergency Care Applied Research Network head injury clinical prediction rules are reliable in practice. Arch Dis Child 2014;99(5):427–31.
19. Bretthauer M, Wieszczy P, Løberg M, et al. Estimated lifetime gained with cancer screening tests: a meta-analysis of randomized clinical trials. JAMA Intern Med 2023;183(11):1196–203.
20. James JT. A new, evidence-based estimate of patient harms associated with hospital care. J Patient Saf 2013;9(3):122–8, 23860193 19. Gilbert EH, Lowenstein SR, Koziol-McLain.
21. Katz ED. Defensive medicine: a case and review of its status and possible solutions. Clin Pract Cases Emerg Med 2019;3(4):329–32.
22. Rothberg MB, Class J, Bishop TF, et al. The cost of defensive medicine on 3 hospital medicine services. JAMA Intern Med 2014;174(11):1867–8.
23. Mello MM, Chandra A, Gawande AA, et al. National costs of the medical liability system. Health Aff 2010;29(9):1569–77.
24. Frakes M, Gruber J. Defensive medicine: evidence from military immunity. Am Econ J Econ Pol 2019;11(3):197–231.
25. Studdert DM, Mello MM, Sage WM, et al. Defensive medicine among high-risk specialist physicians in a volatile malpractice environment. JAMA 2005; 293(21):2609–17.
26. Kanzaria HK, Hoffman JR, Probst MA, et al. Emergency physician perceptions of medically unnecessary advanced diagnostic imaging. Acad Emerg Med 2015; 22(4):390–8.
27. Jena AB, Seabury S, Lakdawalla D, et al. Malpractice risk according to physician specialty. N Engl J Med 2011;365(7):629–36.

28. Seabury SA, Chandra A, Lakdawalla DN, et al. On average, physicians spend nearly 11 percent of their 40-year careers with an open, unresolved malpractice claim. Health Aff 2013;32(1):111–9.

29. Carlson JN, Foster KM, Pines JM, et al. Provider and practice factors associated with emergency physicians' being named in a malpractice claim. Ann Emerg Med 2018;71(2):157–64.e4.

30. Wong KE, Parikh PD, Miller KC, et al. Emergency department and urgent care medical malpractice claims 2001-15. West J Emerg Med 2021;22(2):333–8.

31. Carlson JN, Foster KM, Black BS, et al. Emergency physician practice changes after being named in a malpractice claim. Ann Emerg Med 2020;75(2):221–35.

32. Croskerry P. Achieving quality in clinical decision making: cognitive strategies and detection of bias. Acad Emerg Med 2002;9(11):1184–204.

33. Croskerry P. The importance of cognitive errors in diagnosis and strategies to minimize them. Acad Med 2003;78(8):775–80.

34. Croskerry P. The theory and practice of clinical decision-making. Can J Anesth 2005;52(Suppl 1):R1–8.

35. Laureano-Phillips J, Robinson RD, Aryal S, et al. HEART score risk stratification of low-risk chest pain patients in the emergency department: a systematic review and meta-analysis. Ann Emerg Med 2019;74(2):187–203.

36. Weinstock MB, Weingart S, Orth F, et al. Risk for clinically relevant adverse cardiac events in patients with chest pain at hospital admission. JAMA Intern Med 2015;175(7):1207–12.

37. Spiegel R, Sutherland M, Brown R, et al. Clinically relevant adverse cardiovascular events in intermediate heart score patients admitted to the hospital following a negative emergency department evaluation. Am J Emerg Med 2021;46:469–75.

38. Hess PL, Wojdyla DM, Al-Khatib SM, et al. Sudden cardiac death after non-ST-segment elevation acute coronary syndrome. JAMA Cardiol 2016;1(1):73–9.

39. Peretz A, Dujari S, Cowan R, et al. ACEP Guidelines on Acute Nontraumatic Headache Diagnosis and Management in the Emergency Department, Commentary on Behalf of the Refractory, Inpatient, Emergency Care Section of the American Headache Society. Headache 2020;60(3):643–6.

40. Musey PI Jr, Bellolio F, Upadhye S, et al. Guidelines for reasonable and appropriate care in the emergency department (GRACE): Recurrent, low-risk chest pain in the emergency department. Acad Emerg Med 2021;28(7):718–44.

41. Perry JJ, Sivilotti MLA, Sutherland J, et al. Validation of the Ottawa Subarachnoid Hemorrhage Rule in patients with acute headache [published correction appears in CMAJ. 2018 Feb 12;190(6):E173]. CMAJ (Can Med Assoc J) 2017;189(45): E1379–85.

42. Probst MA, Kanzaria HK, Frosch DL, et al. Perceived appropriateness of shared decision-making in the emergency department: a survey study. Acad Emerg Med 2016;23(4):375–81.

43. Probst MA, Kanzaria HK, Schoenfeld EM, et al. Shared decision making in the emergency department: a guiding framework for clinicians. Ann Emerg Med 2017;70(5): 688–95.

44. Frosch DL, Kaplan RM. Shared decision making in clinical medicine: past research and future directions. Am J Prev Med 1999;17(4):285–94.

45. Schoenfeld EM, Mader S, Houghton C, et al. The effect of shared decision making on patients' likelihood of filing a complaint or lawsuit: a simulation study. Ann Emerg Med 2019;74(1):126–36.

46. Kline JA, Courtney DM, Kabrhel C, et al. Prospective multicenter evaluation of the pulmonary embolism rule-out criteria. J Thromb Haemostasis 2008;6(5):772–80.

Medical Malpractice Epidemiology
Adults and Pediatrics

Kelly Wong Heidepriem, MD*

KEYWORDS

- Malpractice • Medical professional liability • Medicolegal liability
- Emergency medicine malpractice • Pediatric emergency medicine malpractice

KEY POINTS

- There are many factors about the practice and environment of emergency medicine that make practitioners prone to medicolegal risk. By the age of 55 years, 68% of emergency physicians have been sued.
- Reviewing the most common shared factors is of utmost importance for improving patient care and decreasing litigation risk. In adult malpractice claims, the diagnoses that we think of as being high acuity, "can't-miss" diagnoses are also the highest risk for malpractice litigation, including cardiorespiratory arrest, pulmonary embolism, aortic aneurysm, and myocardial infarction.
- Cardiorespiratory arrest also predominates pediatric closed claims, in addition to fractures, appendicitis, respiratory illnesses, and meningitis.

EMERGENCY MEDICINE OVERVIEW

Inherent in emergency medicine (EM) is the routine need to make high-stakes decisions for undifferentiated patients based on limited information. Overcrowding and boarding have become commonplace, but resulting delays in diagnosis and care can lead to poorer outcomes and increased litigation risk.[1,2] Over 90% of physicians in high-risk specialties including EM, change their clinical decision-making due to malpractice risk, a behavior termed "defensive medicine."[3] In addition to the economic impact of malpractice lawsuits, a 2010 estimate suggests that defensive medicine costs approximately US$55 billion per year in the United States[4]; more recent estimates put defensive medicine costs at 2.8% of all health care spending.[5]

In a recent analysis of hospital-based adult malpractice claims, the emergency department (ED) was the third most common origin (9.1%) for a claim, following

Department of Family Medicine, University of South Dakota Sanford School of Medicine, 1400 West 22nd Street, Sioux Falls, SD 57105, USA
* Corresponding author.
E-mail address: wellykong@gmail.com

Emerg Med Clin N Am 43 (2025) 19–28
https://doi.org/10.1016/j.emc.2024.05.018   emed.theclinics.com
0733-8627/25/© 2024 Elsevier Inc. All rights are reserved, including those for text and data mining, AI training, and similar technologies.

operating rooms (40.7%) and inpatient rooms (15.8%).[6] In a poignant letter to the editor, the authors opine that the ED is the safety net not only for the health care system but also for attribution of malpractice. An study in the National Health System found that only approximately half of the claims originating in the ED were attributable to EM providers "and that litigation allocated to the ED is not the same as litigation generated by EM clinicians."[7]

Of physicians of all specialties, emergency physicians (EPs) were more likely to have been sued in their career to date than every nonsurgical specialty in addition to dermatology, ophthalmology, otolaryngology, and urology.[8] A survey of physicians in non-EM specialties found that 39% "definitely will/already decided to" avoid involvement of care for high-risk patients; EPs, however, are unable to choose their patient population. Perhaps, to compensate, more EPs are more likely to report overordering of tests not clinically indicated (70%) compared to physicians in other specialties (59%).[3] Over 60% of EPs reported that their most recent act of defensive medicine was ordering imaging (computed tomography [CT], MRI, or radiograph).[3]

How Many Emergency Physicians Are Sued by the Age of 55 Years?

This malpractice risk remains front of mind for most EPs, and not without cause—nearly 68% over the age of 55 years have been named in a malpractice claim.[8] In those aged under 55 years, approximately 35% of EPs have been named in a lawsuit.[8] About 46.8% of all EPs had been sued in the career to date compared to 31.2% of physicians in all specialties.[7] About 3.3% of EPs reported having been sued in the past year,[8] although this has been quoted as being as high as 7.5% in other studies.[9] There is approximately a 1.5% annual risk of a claim being paid either through settlement or verdict on behalf of an EP.[9]

What Is the Expected Claim Length?

In addition to claim frequency, claim length has consequences for both plaintiffs and defendants. Plaintiffs may face a delay in compensation and both parties may be subject to loss of work in addition to emotional repercussions of a protracted resolution. On average, it takes approximately 15 months for a claim to be filed after an ED visit,[10,11] with an average open claim length between 16.7[10] and 23 months.[11] All-specialty claims with emotional injury take approximately 13.5 months to resolve, compared to claims as a result of fatality or permanent injury that took 22.3 months to resolve.[10] For all specialties, around half of claims that resolved without a payment took more than 1 year; pediatrics and obstetrics had the longest average claim length likely due to their shared involvement of pediatric plaintiffs; this may apply to EPs caring for pediatric patients as well.[10]

In a study reviewing adult malpractice claims, the hospital system was named as a codefendant more often in claims involving EPs (72%) compared to internists (40%) or general surgeons (48%).[11] Nurses were rarely named as codefendants (4%).[11]

Most studies have found that inflation-adjusted indemnity amounts in EM are increasing over time,[11,12] which is consistent with data in an all-specialty study, which reached the same conclusion.[13,14] There is less agreement on whether claim frequency is trending up[11] or down.[13,14]

The American College of Emergency Physicians (ACEP) endorses tort reform including but not limited to caps on noneconomic damages, reduction in term length in statutes of limitation, qualifications for expert witnesses, apologies without admissibility, and recognition of local standards of care in rural areas.[15] ACEP further recommends that following clinical guidelines may reduce litigation risk, citing that OBGYNs who did not follow clinical guidelines and who were 6 times more likely to be sued.[16]

Emergency Physician-Specific Practice Factors

In a study of nearly over 9 million ED visits examining factors associated with being named in a lawsuit, only the total number of years in practice (increasing total number of years in practice) and higher visit volume were statistically significant.[17] Other factors such as board certification (American Board of Emergency Medicine vs American Osteopathic Board of Emergency Medicine), nocturnists, Relative Value Units (RVUs) per hour, Press Ganey percentile, admission rate, working at multiple sites, and state malpractice environment (as rated from a 2014 ACEP report card) were not associated with being named in lawsuits.[17]

In a study analyzing the association between patient satisfaction scores with patient complaints and risk management episodes (meaning "reportable incidents that could lead to a lawsuit, 180 day intention to file letters/threats to file a lawsuit, and attorneys' requests for medical records"), EPs who were in the lowest quartile of patient satisfaction were 2 times more likely to have a complaint. Patient satisfaction with provider was not related to risk management episodes. Those who received greater than 2 complaints per quarter were 4 times more likely to have a risk management episode.[18] There are similar findings reported among inpatient clinicians.[19]

A study of EPs named in a lawsuit showed no change in RVUs per hour or per visit, length of stay, or admission rates in the 4 months before being named in a lawsuit compared to the 4 months after being named. Interestingly, EPs had a 6.5% increase in Press Ganey scores after being named in a lawsuit.[20]

Nonemergency Medicine Factors

We may be able to decrease our malpractice risk by examining risk factors from other specialties. Research has highlighted the importance of the physician–patient communication factors in lawsuit risk. Primary care physicians (PCPs) who had no lawsuits spent longer in visits, set expectations about the flow of a visit, used humor more, and inquired about patients' opinions and understanding compared to PCPs who had been named in a malpractice claim. Of note, the difference in visit length was only 3 minutes.[21]

Practice type and location may also have a bearing on risk, apart from all clinical practice patterns. Physicians who listed their current employment status as independent contractors were more likely to have been sued in their career (36.2%) compared to employees (28.7%); however, this is not necessarily representative of claims that occurred during that employment type.[8] Physicians practicing in the Middle Atlantic region of the country (New Jersey, New York, Pennsylvania) were the most likely to report having been sued in the past year (3.8%) followed by New England (Connecticut, Maine, Massachusetts, New Hampshire, Rhode Island, Vermont; 2.7%), and West North Central (Iowa, Kansas, Minnesota, Missouri, Nebraska, North Dakota, South Dakota; 2.0%). The 3 regions of the country least likely to report having been sued in the past year were East South Central (Alabama, Kentucky, Mississippi, Tennessee; 0.7%), Mountain (Arizona, Colorado, Idaho, New Mexico, Montana, Utah, Nevada, Wyoming; 0.7%), and East North Central (Indiana, Illinois, Michigan, Ohio, Wisconsin; 1.5%).[8]

Diagnostic Errors

Failure-to-diagnosis remains the leading cause in most EM[1,6,11,12,22–26] and non-EM studies.[13,27,28] One analysis found that payments related to errors in diagnosis in all specialties increased by 31.2% over a 12 year study period.[13] A study comparing

EPs with internists and general surgeons found that diagnosis-related errors in adult patients were more common among EPs (58%) compared to internists (42%) and general surgeons (11%).[11] When an error in diagnosis was made in the ED, an adverse outcome was identified in 65% of claims. No adverse outcome was identified in 3% of claims, which highlights the frustration felt by patients receiving incorrect diagnoses who still filed lawsuits despite no adverse result.[23]

A study examining the types of diagnostic error in claims originating from the ED found that the leading associated diagnoses were fractures (19%), infections (15%), myocardial infarction (10%), and cancer (9%). These errors were attributed to EPs 52% of the time, followed by general internists (28%) and surgeons (20%). The median delay in diagnosis was 2.5 days. Trainees were involved in 56% of ED claims with missed diagnoses but this does not always mean that trainees are conamed as defendants. A review of all-specialty claims from the National Practitioner Data Bank between 1991 and 2003 involved a resident trainee less than 1% of the time, with a decrease over the study period from 1.5% at the start to 0.6% by the end.[29]

Further analysis found failure to order tests (58%), inadequate medical history and physical examination (42%), incorrect interpretation of tests (37%), and failure to request a consultation (33%) were the most common factors contributing to resulting errors in diagnosis.[23] Of the tests not ordered that would have improved the patient's clinical course, plain radiographs (22%), CT (17%), cardiac enzyme tests (15%), ultrasound (13%), and hematologic laboratory tests (11%) were the most common.[23] However, even tests ordered can be misinterpreted. Of tests that were incorrectly interpreted, EPs were responsible for misinterpretation 48% of the time, and radiology was responsible 41% of the time. Plain radiographs were the test most likely to be misinterpreted (66%). This may be the result of many EPs having to self-interpret in the absence of real-time plain radiograph reads by radiology.[23] Electrocardiograms (EKGs) were the culprit in 10% of misinterpreted tests.[23]

Point-of-Care Ultrasound

Two main studies examining legal risk and point-of-care ultrasound (POCUS). The first reviewed lawsuits found in Westlaw from 2008 to 2012 and found that 5 lawsuits involved POCUS. In 3 of the cases, the plaintiff alleged that the POCUS study was within the scope of the EPs' practice; in the 2 remaining cases, the plaintiff alleged a delay or error in testing being performed by the radiology department.[30] A separate study reviewed a different legal database from 2011 to 2021 and found 10 claims involving POCUS in emergency settings. Seven of these cases involved pediatrics. One lawsuit claimed the wrong ultrasound study was initially performed, and another case was based on improper diagnosis made after an ultrasound. The remaining 8 lawsuits centered around failure to consider a diagnosis (most commonly appendicitis or testicular torsion) and/or failure to order an ultrasound.[31]

The allegation of failure to perform POCUS when it is within the EPs scope as a basis for lawsuits may increase in the coming years, due to many recently trained EM physicians graduating with a letter stating that they have satisfied their residency's POCUS training requirements.

ADULT MALPRACTICE CLAIMS

In recent studies of EM claims in adult patients, approximately two-thirds of malpractice lawsuits are dropped, withdrawn, or dismissed.[6] An additional 23% of claims are settled with an average indemnity of US$297,709.[6] Of lawsuits that ultimately go to trial, the defendant won 92.6% of the time. In the 7.4% of cases where the verdict was found for the plaintiff, average indemnity was US$816,909. Defense fees for trials were US$111,446 when juries found in favor of the defense and US$159,716 when juries found in favor of the plaintiff.[6] Average defense fees for dropped/withdrawn/dismissed lawsuits in closed adult EM claims are slightly lower at US$22,996 compared to settled claims (US$55,260), perhaps accounted for by the shorter average claim length of the former.[6]

Other EM studies that do not break down by specific claim outcome (ie, dropped/dismissed/withdrawn vs jury verdict vs settled) find that approximately 24% to 31% resulted in a verdict/settlement payment to the plaintiff[11,13]; the median indemnity in one study was US$206,261.[11]

The percentage breakdown in claim outcome has remained relatively stable over time. A commonly referenced prior dataset of EM data from 1985 to 2007 found 64% of claims were dropped/withdrawn/dismissed, 29% settled, and 7% went to trial.[12] In the Brown dataset, juries ruled in favor of EPs 85% of the time.[12] These data are also very similar to all-specialty data: A study from the American Medical Association found that for all specialties between 2016 and 2018, 65% of claims were dropped, withdrawn, or dismissed, 6% of claims went to trial with a verdict in favor of the defendant 89% of the time.[8]

High-Risk Diagnoses (Adults)

Cardiac/cardiorespiratory arrest, pulmonary embolism, aortic aneurysms, acute myocardial infarction, fractures, and infections are consistently some of the highest risk diagnoses in adult closed claims.[6,11,23] One recent study found the breakdown to be cardiac or cardiorespiratory arrest (9.1%), acute myocardial infarction (4.0%), aortic aneurysm (2.3%), pulmonary embolism (2.2%), and appendicitis (2.0%).[6] The diagnosis with the highest average indemnity was aortic aneurysms with an average indemnity of US$369,872.[6]

Of the aforementioned diagnoses, acute myocardial infarction was the most likely to result in a payment (39%) with an average indemnity of US$306,487.[6] Nationally, there are around 7 million ED visits for chest pain each year. Reynolds and colleagues estimated that ST-elevation myocardial infarction (STEMI) incidence decreased almost 9% per year between 2000 and 2008.[32] The overall incidence of STEMIs is decreasing, likely in part due to the advancement of modern cardiovascular medicine including statins, aggressive cardioprotective recommendations for blood pressure and cholesterol, stress tests, and angiography.[32] An older study in the EM literature found that around 6% of ST elevation cases were misinterpreted by EPs.[33] For more on chest pain-specific legal risk, refer to the article by Dr Matt Delaney.

In 25% of claims, procedural complications are cited, most commonly intubation (7%), suturing (5%), and lumbar punctures (3%). Of these, intubation resulted in the highest indemnity payments (median US$308,970).[11]

Severity of Injury (Adults)

Death is the most commonly cited outcome listed in malpractice claims,[6,11,12] but grave/permanent injury is most likely to result in a payment[11,12] (29.5% vs 32%).[6] A paid claim resulting in death on average pays out US$326,350, which is less than half the average indemnity for a claim resulting in grave injury (US$686,239).[6] The higher average indemnity is usually related to ongoing economic damages and ongoing costs of medical care. Lawsuits claiming minor or major permanent injury resulted in average indemnities of US$248,662 to US$505,965 and claims resulting in minor or major temporary injury resulted in indemnities of US$152,910 to US$215,244.[6] Emotional damage or legal issues tend to make up less than 10% of total claims[11,12] and only resulted in a payment to the plaintiff around 10% of the time.[12]

Cited Contributing Factors (Adults)

As previously mentioned, multiple data sets analyzing closed malpractice claims in EM found that errors in diagnosis consistently remains the top cited reason for malpractice litigation.[6,11,12,23] In a recent comprehensive study, errors in diagnosis comprised "36.4% of closed claims, followed by improper performance (17.7%), failure to supervise or monitor case (5.2%); and medication errors (3.4%)."[6]

Failure to supervise or monitor case

It is anticipated that advanced practice providers may be the primary caregivers for 20% of total ED visits by 2030.[34] For EPs who may be supervising nurse practitioners (NPs), physician assistants (PAs), or may be cosigning their notes without interacting with the patient, this is of particular interest. In a study by Antkowiak and colleagues reviewing over 5000 closed claims, 3.3% involved an NP, 8.8% involved a PA, and 9.2% involved a trainee.[35] Similarly, Myers and colleagues found that 7% of adult closed claims involved a physician trainee.[11] Average indemnity for diagnosis-related claim was higher for trainee-related cases (US$856,378) compared to NPs (US$411,988), PAs (US$580,664), or nontrainee EPs (US$497,264). The Antkowiak and colleagues study found that claims involving trainees were statistically more likely to involve errors in diagnosis.[35]

For more on legal risk to the resident in training (and attending), see the following article by Dr Nicole Tyczynska and Dr Rebecca Younker. For more on collaboration of physicians and PAs and NPs, refer to the following article by Dr Kimberly Bambach.

PEDIATRIC MALPRACTICE CLAIMS

Pediatric patients pose diagnostic challenges for many reasons that do not exist in the average adult patient. For example, neonates and infants cannot yet talk, and children might not yet possess the vocabulary to explain their symptoms. Shyness or a lack of understanding may lead even teenagers to shirk away from complaints that they find embarrassing (ie, testicular or pelvic pain). Physicians have been trained to prioritize conservative care in pediatric patients, for example, reducing our use of radiating imaging or ordering fewer laboratory studies compared to our average adult workup for similar complaints.[36,37]

Similarly, the legal environment surrounding pediatrics is as different as the clinical environment is. While the statute of limitations in adults for most states is 2 years (although in some states can be up to 5 years) from the time of alleged malpractice,[38] there is incredible state-to-state variability in statute of limitations for pediatric plaintiffs. One medicolegal review found that for newborn patients, the statute of limitations ranges from 1 up to 23 years,[38] well past the age of majority in most states. Additionally, there is a longer potential lifetime of a pediatric plaintiff compared to an adult plaintiff, resulting in higher calculated economic damages, lost potential wages, or ongoing medical expenses.[39]

In general, pediatricians have a very low malpractice risk compared to EPs. When pediatric claims do occur, however, most originate in the ED[37] and the average indemnity for pediatric lawsuits is 60% more than the average for all claims.[39] There currently exist 2 comprehensive studies reviewing pediatric malpractice claims in recent years using a similar source but from different years.[24,26]

In the most recent comprehensive analysis of pediatric malpractice claims by Glerum and colleagues, a payment to the plaintiff was made in 30% of cases, with an average of US$319,513.[26] Approximately 87% of closed pediatric claims are dropped, withdrawn, or dismissed. This rate is lower than in an older study in pediatrics (92%).[24]

This is also significantly higher than the rate at which adult claims are dropped, withdrawn, or dismissed (65.9%).[6] Only 8% of claims went to trial in the Glerum study,[26] which is consistent over time compared to the Selbst data (7%).[24] Overall, when cases went to a jury trial, verdicts were still more likely to favor the defendant (82%),[26] but at a lower rate than in cases involving adult patients (92.6%).[6]

In all pediatric claims that originated from either emergency or urgent care centers, EPs were named in 38.9% of closed claims, followed by pediatrics (13%), family practice (12.4%), orthopedic surgery (8.2%), and radiology (6.3%). Of these specialties, radiology was the specialty that, if named, was most likely to result in a payment to a plaintiff (41.3% of the time). When EPs were named in case, 31.1% of the closed claims resulted in an indemnity payment.[26]

High-Risk Diagnoses (Pediatrics)

Pediatrics has had a notable shift in most commonly cited diagnoses in closed claims. Historically, meningitis reigned as one of the more common cited diagnoses in almost every age group.[37] In the past 2 decades, cardiac or cardiorespiratory arrest has replaced it to become the diagnosis most likely to result in a claim, with the exception of fractures in the 12 to 17 year age range.[37] Meningitis has either fallen down the list as less likely or fallen off the top diagnoses completely.[37] Glerum and colleagues found the highest risk diagnoses listed in closed claims to be cardiac or cardiorespiratory arrest (11.4%), appendicitis (4.1%), disorder of male genital organs (4.0%), encephalopathy not further defined (3.4%), and meningitis (2.6%).[26]

Appendicitis consistently remains a common diagnosis of concern.[24,26,37] It is the second most commonly cited diagnosis in every age group over 3 years old.[37] However, in patients aged under 3 years, respiratory diagnoses like diseases of the lung are more likely to be cited than appendicitis.[37]

For further information on high-risk pediatric conditions, refer to the article by Dr Ilene Claudius.

Severity of injury (pediatrics)

Thirty-one percentage of claims involved a patient death, but—consistent with the adult literature—major permanent injury (46.7) or grave injury (38.9%) was more likely to result in a payment to the plaintiff.[26] In claims that resulted in a death, 28.6% resulted in an indemnity payment to plaintiffs.[26] Average indemnity for death was US$249,208, for grave injury was US$923,655, and for major permanent injury was US$551,500.[26] Of interest, only 1.4% of claims were for emotional injury only, and resulted in zero paid claims.[26]

Cited contributing factors (pediatrics)

Similar to adult EM closed claims as well as closed claims from other specialties, errors in diagnosis were the most common cited factor,[24,26] identified in 41.5% of closed pediatric claims.[26] It was cited in over half (50.9%) of paid claims. Improper performance was in cited in 19.9% of paid claims, followed by delay in performance (5.5%), failure to recognize a complication of a treatment (4.5%).[26] Failure or delay in admission to the hospital, despite being much less frequently cited at eighth place, had the highest average indemnity at US$942,500.[26] Medication errors are oft-discussed—especially with pediatrics and weight-based dosing—but only accounted for 3.2% of closed claims and 1.8% of paid claims.[26] The factor that was most likely to result in a payment to the plaintiff was "failure to recognize a complication of treatment," which when cited resulted in a payment 43.5% of the time.[26]

SUMMARY

The following articles delve into the topics such as documentation tips, high-risk diagnoses, managing litigation stress, and many others. We sincerely hope that the information results not only in the improvement of patient care but also in decreased litigation risk.

CLINICS CARE POINTS

- Nearly 68% of EPs over the age of 55 years have been named in malpractice claim. In those aged under 55 years, approximately 35% of emergency physicians have been named in a lawsuit.
- Cardiac/cardiorespiratory arrest, pulmonary embolisms, aortic aneurysms, acute myocardial infarctions, fractures, and infections are amongst the highest risk diagnoses for resulting litigation.
- In a recent study of adult malpractice claims, approximatley two-thirds of lawsuits are dropped, withdrawn, or dismissed.
- Of lawsuits in adult patients that go to trial, juries find in favor of the defendant 92.6% of the time.

DISCLOSURE

The authors have nothing to disclose.

REFERENCES

1. Fordyce J, Blank FS, Pekow P, et al. Errors in a busy emergency department. Ann Emerg Med 2003;42(3):324–33.
2. Biros MH, Adams JG, Wears RL. Errors in emergency medicine: a call to action. Acad Emerg Med 2000;7(11):1173–4.
3. Studdert DM, Mello MM, Sage WM, et al. Defensive medicine among high-risk specialist physicians in a volatile malpractice environment. JAMA 2005;293(21): 2609–17.
4. Mello MM, Chandra A, Gawande AA, et al. National costs of the medical liability system. Health Aff 2010;29(9):1569–77.
5. Katz ED. Defensive medicine: a case and review of its status and possible solutions. Clin Pract Cases Emerg Med 2019;3(4):329–32. PMID: 31763580; PMCID: PMC6861029.
6. Wong KE, Parikh PD, Miller KC, et al. Emergency department and urgent care medical malpractice claims 2001-15. West J Emerg Med 2021;22(2): 333–8.
7. Price J, Barnard EBG, Selway J, et al. The emergency department or the emergency medicine service? Redefining the boundaries of responsibility for emergency care litigation in England. Emerg Med J 2023;40(10):698–9.
8. Guardado. Medical liability claim frequency among U.S. Physicians. American Medical Association Policy Research Perspectives, Available at: https://www.ama-assn.org/system/files/policy-research-perspective-medical-liability-claim-frequency.pdf. Accessed April 1, 2024.
9. Jena AB, Seabury S, Lakdawalla D, et al. Malpractice risk according to physician specialty. N Engl J Med 2011;365(7):629–36.

10. Seabury SA, Chandra A, Lakdawalla DN, et al. On average, physicians spend nearly 11 percent of their 40-year careers with an open, unresolved malpractice claim. Health Aff 2013;32(1):111–9.

11. Myers LC, Einbinder J, Camargo CA Jr, et al. Characteristics of medical malpractice claims involving emergency medicine physicians. J Healthc Risk Manag 2021;41(1):9–15.

12. Brown TW, McCarthy ML, Kelen GD, et al. An epidemiologic study of closed emergency department malpractice claims in a national database of physician malpractice insurers. Acad Emerg Med 2010;17(5):553–60.

13. Gupta A, Snyder A, Kachalia A, et al. Malpractice claims related to diagnostic errors in the hospital. BMJ Qual Saf 2017.

14. Schaffer AC, Jena AB, Seabury SA, et al. Rates and Characteristics of Paid Malpractice Claims Among US Physicians by Specialty, 1992-2014. JAMA Intern Med 2017;177(5):710–8.

15. Reform of Tort Law. American College of Emergency Physicians Policy Statement. Available at: https://www.acep.org/patient-care/policy-statements/reform-of-tort-law. [Accessed 31 January 2024].

16. Ransom SB, Studdert DM, Dombrowski MP, et al. Reduced medicolegal risk by compliance with obstetric clinical pathways: a case–control study. Obstet Gynecol 2003;101(4):751–5.

17. Carlson JN, Foster KM, Pines JM, et al. Provider and practice factors associated with emergency physicians' being named in a malpractice claim. Ann Emerg Med 2018;71(2):157–64.e4.

18. Cydulka RK, Tamayo-Sarver J, Gage A, et al. Association of patient satisfaction with complaints and risk management among emergency physicians. J Emerg Med 2011;41(4):405–11.

19. Stelfox HT, Gandhi TK, Orav EJ, et al. The relation of patient satisfaction with complaints against physicians and malpractice lawsuits. Am J Med 2005;118(10):1126–33.

20. Carlson JN, Foster KM, Black BS, et al. Emergency physician practice changes after being named in a malpractice claim. Ann Emerg Med 2020;75(2):221–35.

21. Levinson W, Roter DL, Mullooly JP, et al. Physician-patient communication. The relationship with malpractice claims among primary care physicians and surgeons. JAMA 1997;277(7):553–9.

22. Gupta K, Szymonifka J, Rivadeneira NA, et al. Factors associated with malpractice claim payout: an analysis of closed emergency department claims. Joint Comm J Qual Patient Saf 2022;48(9):492–5.

23. Kachalia A, Gandhi TK, Puopolo AL, et al. Missed and delayed diagnoses in the emergency department: a study of closed malpractice claims from 4 liability insurers. Ann Emerg Med 2007;49(2):196–205.

24. Selbst SM, Friedman MJ, Singh SB. Epidemiology and etiology of malpractice lawsuits involving children in US emergency departments and urgent care centers. Pediatr Emerg Care 2005;21(3):165–9.

25. White AA, Wright SW, Blanco R, et al. Cause-and-effect analysis of risk management files to assess patient care in the emergency department. Acad Emerg Med 2004;11(10):1035–41.

26. Glerum KM, Selbst SM, Parikh PD, et al. Pediatric malpractice claims in the emergency department and urgent care settings from 2001 to 2015. Pediatr Emerg Care 2021;37(7):e376–9.

27. Phillips RL Jr, Bartholomew LA, Dovey SM, et al. Learning from malpractice claims about negligent, adverse events in primary care in the United States. Qual Saf Health Care 2004;13(2):121–6.

28. Chandra A, Nundy S, Seabury SA. The growth of physician medical malpractice payments: evidence from the National Practitioner Data Bank. Health Aff 2005;(Suppl Web Exclusives):W5–249.

29. Kachalia A, Studdert DM. Professional liability issues in graduate medical education. JAMA 2004;292(9):1051–6.

30. Stolz L, O'Brien KM, Miller ML, et al. A review of lawsuits related to point-of-care emergency ultrasound applications. West J Emerg Med 2015;16(1):1–4.

31. Solomon L, Emma M, Gibbons LM, et al. Current risk landscape of point-of-care ultrasound in pediatric emergency medicine in medical malpractice litigation. Am J Emerg Med 2022;58:16–21.

32. Reynolds K, Go AS, Leong TK, et al. Trends in incidence of hospitalized acute myocardial infarction in the cardiovascular research network (CVRN). Am J Med 2017;130(3):317–27.

33. Brady WJ, Perron A, Ullman E. Errors in emergency physician interpretation of ST-segment elevation in emergency department chest pain patients. Acad Emerg Med 2000;7(11):1256–60.

34. Marco CA, Courtney DM, Ling LJ, et al. The emergency medicine physician workforce: projections for 2030. Ann Emerg Med 2021;78(6):726–37.

35. Antkowiak PS, Lai SY, Burke RC, et al. Characterizing malpractice cases involving emergency department advanced practice providers, physicians in training, and attending physicians. Acad Emerg Med 2023;30(12):1237–45.

36. Weinstock MB, Jolliff H. High-risk medicolegal conditions in pediatric emergency medicine. Emerg Med Clin North Am 2021;39(3):479–91.

37. Edwards BL, Dorfman D. High-risk pediatric emergencies. Emerg Med Clin North Am 2020;38(2):383–400.

38. Shea KG, Scanlan KJ, Nilsson KJ, et al. Interstate variability of the statute of limitations for medical liability: a cause for concern? J Pediatr Orthop 2008;28(3):370–4.

39. AAP Department of Practice, Pediatric malpractice claims low in frequency but high in severity, *AAP News*, 35 (1), 2014, 22.

Medicolegally Protective Documentation in Emergency Medicine

Michael Pallaci, DO[a,b,c,d,e,*], Kevin Markowski, MD[a,d,e], Brock Landrum, MD[a,e]

KEYWORDS

- Emergency medicine • Documentation • Malpractice • Medicolegal • Charting

KEY POINTS

- Medical documentation is directed at three audiences for three distinct purposes: other caregivers for continuity of care, billers and coders for reimbursement, and juries/attorneys for medicolegal protection.
- The most effective way to decrease the likelihood of a lawsuit being filed and of an adverse judgment if to be filed is to effectively communicate the thought process behind clinical decision making, both to patients and to families at the bedside and in the chart.
- The most critical areas of the chart for medicolegal defense are the History of Present Illness (HPI), Medical Decision Making (MDM), and Discharge Instructions.
- Optimally, charting should be done in real time to optimize efficiency and accuracy. At minimum, the HPI and MDM should be completed at the time of service, with the MDM section being used as a "hard stop" to assure that the clinical decisions made during the course of the patient's care are justified by the charting.

INTRODUCTION
Background

Medical documentation is directed at three audiences for three distinct purposes.[1] First and foremost is communication with other health care professionals to communicate the thought process of the clinician and clinical impression, and to facilitate continuity

[a] Northeast Ohio Medical University, 4209 State Route 44, Rootstwon, OH 44272, USA; [b] Ohio University Heritage College of Osteopathic Medicine, 191 West Union Street, Athens, OH 45701, USA; [c] Virtual Care Simulation Lab, Emergency Medicine Residency Program, Department of Emergency Medicine, Summa Health System, 141 North Forge Street, Akron, OH 44303, USA; [d] US Acute Care Solutions, 4535 Dressler Road Northwest, Canton, OH 44718, USA; [e] Department of Emergency Medicine, Summa Health System, 151 North Forge Street, Akron, OH 44303, USA
* Corresponding author. Department of Emergency Medicine, Summa Health System, 151 North Forge Street, Akron, OH 44304.
E-mail address: pallacim@usacs.com
Twitter: @MikePallaci (M.P.); @DrMarkowski (K.M.)

Emerg Med Clin N Am 43 (2025) 29–40
https://doi.org/10.1016/j.emc.2024.05.019
emed.theclinics.com

of care. The second audience is billers and coders for the purpose of reimbursement. In this article, we focus on the third of these purposes, the documentation of clinical findings, decision-making process, and clinical course for medicolegal protection.

In 2011, Jena and colleagues[2] reported that more than 75% of emergency physicians will be named in a malpractice suit at some point in their careers. By the time a physician is questioned by a lawyer at deposition and eventually in front of a jury, significant time will have passed and details of the encounter will have been forgotten. The chart, not the physician's recollection of events, is the primary source of information that will reflect the encounter and determine the outcome. Many physicians try to mitigate medicolegal risk by ordering more tests, admitting more patients to the hospital, and/or referring to more specialists.[3,4] Although these interventions add significant time and cost to the patient encounter, they do little to decrease liability. In fact, there is general agreement among those who defend physicians in lawsuits that the best way to avoid a malpractice action is to spend more time with patients, improve communication, and effectively convey our thought process, both with patients and with families at the bedside and in the medical record.[5,6]

In a 30-year career, the average clinical emergency physician will see more than 100,000 patients. It is not realistic to expect to proactively identify which one or two of these 100,000 patient interactions might land us in court, so documenting each case appropriately is critical. It is important to remember that our role in documenting the patient encounter is not to act as a scribe or transcriptionist and record every word that the patient says. Our role is to document the story in a way that is internally consistent and that reflects our understanding of the patient's presentation while accurately describing our reasons for the workup and treatments we choose to implement.

History

With a strong push from financial incentives provided by the Centers for Medicare and Medicaid Services in 2009, medical documentation has almost universally moved from paper charting to electronic medical records (EMR). Although there are numerous benefits to this change, the shift has resulted in degradation of provider satisfaction,[7,8] decreased efficiency,[9,10] and (at least during the implementation phase) increased medicolegal risk.[11]

After nearly two decades of experience of using EMR, multiple best practices as well as pitfalls to avoid have been identified, and many of those are discussed in detail in this article. The overriding theme is well summarized in a 2015 position paper from the American College of Physicians, which stated "the primary goal of the electronic health record-generated documentation should be concise, history-rich notes that reflect the information gathered and are used to develop an impression, a diagnostic and/or treatment plan, and recommended follow-up."[12]

DISCUSSION
Key Portions of the Chart from a Medicolegal Perspective

Thorough documentation of the events of the patient's emergency department (ED) course as well as documentation of the thought process of patient's care are core tenets of medicolegal protection. The entire chart will be scrutinized in the event of a bad outcome that leads to legal action. Every section has the potential to contain critical information for the defense or for the plaintiff. Providers frequently use prewritten templates to document the physical examination. This improves efficiency but can lead to omission of detailed examination elements performed when the clinical presentation demands. For example, documenting symmetric radial pulses in a patient with chest pain demonstrates that aortic dissection was considered. Documenting a cranial nerve examination, cerebellar examination, test of skew, and evaluation for nystagmus adds depth to the neurologic examination in a patient with vertigo when compared with a generic templated examination entry, such as "Awake, alert and oriented, moves all extremities equally well, normal speech and mental status." The chart should tell a story: What happened in the ED? What did the patient look like? What made it safe to discharge the patient? What critical diagnoses were considered, and how were they excluded? Why were the tests that were ordered chosen, and why were others not? Although every section of the chart plays a role in telling this story, the most critical sections of the chart to answer these questions and therefore provide legal protection are the History of Present Illness (HPI), Medical Decision Making (MDM), and Discharge Instructions.

The HPI is simply a description of the patient's illness. It will typically address the onset, location, duration, severity and quality of symptoms, any associated signs or symptoms, as well as the context in which they occurred and any alleviating or exacerbating factors. The history is generally documented in the patient's own words where possible, with good descriptors to paint a picture for the reader. A few key points to remember when documenting the HPI include the following:

Providers need to be diligent about reviewing the nurses' notes and addressing any discrepancies, particularly when loaded terms, such as "severe," "lethargic," "worst headache of their life," are used.

Any factors contributing to an incomplete or insufficient history (inability to speak, lack of cooperation/participation in the interview, altered mental status, acuity of patient's presentation, and so forth) should be identified in the chart.

Beware of referring to the patient in terms with negative connotations (ie, obese, disheveled, malodorous, difficult, and so forth) or using the patient's words in quotes, especially if vulgar. Consider the purpose of including these descriptors, and whether there is a net benefit if there is a bad outcome. If these do not further the goal of reaching a diagnosis, then consider omitting. If unsure whether to include it, consider the following question: would it be uncomfortable having to read the chart back to a jury in court?

Incorporating key aspects of the Past Medical History, Social History, Family History, and Review of Systems (ROS) into the HPI can help to illustrate thought process and risk stratification. Of note, many EMRs auto-import much of this information to the patient's record. These auto-imports should be reviewed for accuracy and incorporated into the explanation of the decisions made in the patient's ED management.

Although the use of checkboxes and templates for physical examination documentation can be helpful in terms of efficiency as well as completeness if done properly (see "Templates" in Controversies/Pitfalls section in later discussion), using checkbox formats for other parts of the chart, particularly the HPI and MDM, makes the chart more difficult to read and potentially squanders an opportunity for medicolegal protection by not clearly illustrating the provider's thought process.

As of January 1, 2023, the coding of the chart is based entirely on the MDM section, and requirements for documentation of HPI, ROS, and physical examination elements are no longer required for coding and billing purposes.[13] However, from a medicolegal standpoint, these sections remain critical. For example, a patient dies of pulmonary embolus weeks after being seen in the ED for leg pain that was diagnosed as a muscle strain. If, on the first visit, it is well documented that the patient did not have chest pain, shortness of breath, or tachycardia, that risk factors for deep vein thrombosis (DVT) were not present, and that there were no physical examination findings to suggest DVT, the charting ensures a much better opportunity for defense if litigation occurs.

The MDM documentation is the most important area of the chart to describe the provider's thought process and thus will be the focus if there is a bad outcome and litigation occurs. This is the opportunity for the provider to tell the story of the visit as they saw it, to describe what diagnoses were considered and how they were confirmed or excluded, the rationale for treatments provided or not provided. The clinical course is also described here, including reevaluations; discussions with the patient, family, and/or consultants; and interpretation of diagnostic test results. It is neither useful nor necessary to repeat the HPI or list all test results in the MDM section. It is not a place to contribute to "note bloat" with redundant information, but rather a place to describe how that information was used in decision making.

The MDM section should be completed before disposition. We recommend using it as a "hard stop" before disposition, particularly if the patient is being discharged. It should be used as an opportunity to demonstrate that the disposition decision and the ED care have adequately excluded life-threatening/"can't-miss" diagnoses, and to describe a reassessment of the patient. A careful and through thought process along with communication with the patient and their family, reflected in the documentation, is the most effective way to avoid an adverse judgment or to avoid the lawsuit being filed in the first place.

The MDM section should also include documentation of discussions with the patient and their family regarding any diagnostic uncertainty, as well as which diagnostic tests and therapeutic interventions are being ordered and why. Explaining the provider's thought process encourages the patient and/or family to express additional concerns and add to the history, decreasing the likelihood of a missed diagnosis. In addition, these discussions improve patient and family satisfaction, decreasing the likelihood of a potential lawsuit if a bad outcome eventually occurs. Documentation of these discussions illustrates involvement of the patient in the decision making and illustrates the provider's careful thought process and decreases the likelihood of an adverse judgment if a lawsuit is eventually filed.

A bad outcome is difficult to defend if inadequate discharge instructions were given, or if they were given but not documented in the record. Good discharge instructions include the following elements[1]:

Follow-up instructions should be time specific. In addition, providers should consider including documentation if they spoke to a consultant to facilitate close follow-up ("Call your primary physician today to schedule a follow-up appointment for next week. I spoke with Dr Jones [Urology] from the ED, his office staff will call you to set up an appointment for tomorrow, call him yourself if you have not heard from his office by lunchtime.")

Instructions for medication use, both prescription and over the counter ("Take antibiotics as prescribed until they are gone. Use prescribed naproxen twice daily on a schedule until it is gone, not just as needed. Add over-the-counter acetaminophen 1000 mg up to four times daily as needed for pain.")

Instructions specific to the diagnosis/symptoms ("Rest, ice, and elevate your injured extremity above the level of your heart as much as you can. You can bear weight as tolerated. Use crutches as needed for comfort.")

Return precautions are perhaps the most important part of the discharge instructions from a medicolegal perspective.

List signs and symptoms that specifically apply to their diagnosis and symptoms ("Return to the ED for fever, loss of urine or stool control (incontinence), or inability to pass urine or stool, if unable to use or to feel your legs, if pain is not responding to medications") and then close with a general statement ("...if symptoms persist, change or worsen, or if any other problems arise").

Document scheduled returns in those circumstances where hospitalization is not required but the patient requires closer follow-up than what can realistically be provided on an outpatient basis (abscess or wound rechecks, abdominal pain, and so forth). In these situations, it is common (and medicolegally protective) practice to instruct the patient to return to the ED for reevaluation.

Using a term such as "As discussed in the ED..." in the discharge instructions is recommended to remind the patient and their family of the instructions provided at bedside, as well as to document the conversation ("As discussed in the ED, your CT scan was negative for a blood clot in your lung, but did show a nodule that will need to be monitored to assure no changes over time that would be concerning for cancer. Be sure to discuss this with your primary physician on your follow-up appointment so that repeat imaging can be arranged").

Documentation of Comanagement with Residents/Advance Practice Providers

Many physicians will supervise residents in training as well as advanced practice providers (APPs) in the ED. Every resident patient encounter must be supervised by an attending physician; APPs will see some patients independently and will consult the attending physician when the patient presentation requires it (rules governing these interactions vary by state). When comanaging cases with residents and APPs, the ultimate responsibility for the patient lies with the attending physician. Documentation of comanagement should specify that the attending physician independently evaluated the patient and should contain the important information that contributed to the MDM. Key portions of the history, physical examination, and especially the MDM should be documented independently by the supervising physician rather than depending on the adequacy of the resident or APP documentation. The supervising physician must assure that established supervision policy is followed, and that an internally consistent chart is constructed that depicts a history, physical examination, and workup that is consistent with the documented disposition and follow-up instructions.

Scribes

Scribes are used in many EDs to help with documentation and physician efficiency. Scribes have been shown to increase efficiency by up to 15%,[14] but they are not providers. When a scribe is involved in a patient encounter, the physician is required to affirm that the note accurately documents the information collected and care provided. The chart needs to be carefully examined to assure that this is actually the case, as this will be assumed to be accurate in court. Although the physician should personally document the MDM and discharge instructions when working with a scribe, the HPI will be documented by the scribe.

Informed Consent/Decision-Making Capacity

The Joint Commission provides the following definition of informed consent: "Agreement or permission accompanied by full notice about the care, treatment, or service that is the subject of the consent. A patient must be apprised of the nature, risks, and alternatives of a medical procedure or treatment before the physician or other health care professional begins any such course. After receiving this information, the patient then either consents to or refuses such a procedure or treatment."[15] (See also chapter 5: Informed Consent and EMTALA—Procedural and AMA.)

Informed consent is a process of communication as opposed to simply a signature on a piece of paper. The nature of the procedure/treatment, as well as the risks, benefits, and alternatives should be documented. Although a signed form is not always required for adequate documentation of informed consent, it provides an extra layer of confirmation that consent was provided.

Capacity Versus Competency

The documentation must include the patient's capacity to make medical decisions. It is important to distinguish between *competency*, a legal term determined by a court, and decision-making *capacity*, a medical term determined by a physician. A "power of attorney" only becomes applicable in situations when the patient is unable to make decisions for themselves (ie, lacks decision-making capacity). Appropriate documentation of this determination includes the patient's ability to understand and process the information presented (ideally repeating it back in their own words), to understand the weight and gravity of the decision, and to clearly communicate a choice.[16]

In situations where informed consent cannot be obtained (ie, an unresponsive patient requiring an emergent intervention with no designated power of attorney available) and/or in cases when the patient lacks decision-making capacity, the concept of emergency implied consent is applied. In this case, adequate documentation includes an explanation of the urgency of the intervention and of the reason the physician thinks that the patient cannot provide informed consent, and a statement of the belief that a prudent person in a similar circumstance would consent to the intervention.

Shared Decision Making

Dr Erik Hess defines shared decision making (SDM) as "a collaborative process in which patients and providers make health care decisions together, taking into account the best scientific evidence available, as well as the patient's values and preferences."[17] SDM involves the discussion of 2 or more approaches to diagnosis or treatment that the clinician considers to be reasonable. For example, SDM would be appropriate when deciding whether to obtain a head CT after a minor head injury, but not appropriate when discussing why it would not be reasonable for a patient with pneumonia, hypoxia, tachycardia, and an acute kidney injury to be discharged.

Documentation of SDM is more involved than simply stating that it happened. Important elements of SDM documentation include that the patient or surrogate decision maker has decision-making capacity, that there was ample opportunity for discussion and questions, which approaches were discussed, what guidance was provided by the physician, and that specific data were shared in layman's terms and understood by the people involved in the decision. For example, "I participated in a shared decision making process with the patient and his wife regarding the disposition decision. We discussed his risk stratification (HEART score of 4) and the available morbidity and mortality data. This information was presented in layman's terms. We discussed the risks and benefits of the available options, specifically hospital observation versus discharge with close outpatient cardiology follow-up. The patient and his wife participated actively in the discussion and asked multiple questions, which I was able to answer for them. They clearly understood the information presented. Their preference was for outpatient management. I was able to obtain a cardiology appointment for them in 2 days. Return precautions were provided at bedside as well as in the discharge instructions."

Informed Refusal

A patient may decline a test or treatment option recommended by a caregiver. In contrast to SDM, where the caregiver's preference may be different than the patient's but both are considered safe and reasonable, these are situations where one option is considered demonstrably superior by the treating physician but the patient or their decision maker declines to accept this recommendation.

If the patient or their decision maker declines an intervention recommended by the provider after a discussion of the risks and benefits, they are making an informed refusal of care. The important components of documentation for informed refusal are similar to those for informed consent and for SDM.

Against Medical Advice

If the intervention that the patient is refusing is hospital admission and the risk of a patient refusing care is substantial, the provider should document that the patient is acting against medical advice (AMA). In both of these scenarios, it is important to provide the patient with the best management that they agree to (antibiotics for outpatient treatment of infections, adequate analgesia and symptom management, referrals for close follow-up, including with specialists if indicated, and so forth).

AMA documentation should include an indication that efforts were undertaken to make sure that the patient understood the risks, that they were adamant in their refusal, and that they were encouraged to return if they changed their mind.

Hospitals may require that an AMA form be signed despite the lack of significant medicolegal protection that it provides. Although there is some controversy on this topic, it is of little consequence, as there is no downside to the form being signed. Regardless, it is the opinion of these authors that clear documentation of the discussion with the patient and of the elements discussed above and not the signature on the AMA form will provide medicolegal protection if a bad outcome occurs. The discharge process should mirror any other discharge, with adequate discharge instructions and outpatient treatment/referrals provided. In addition to documentation in the MDM section of the chart, it is important to include these elements for the patient in their discharge instructions. For example, "As discussed in the ED, you are leaving against my advice prior to completion of your evaluation and treatment for your myocardial infarction (heart attack). By doing so, you are putting yourself at risk for the complications of an untreated heart attack, which include but are not limited to further damage to heart muscle and associated heart failure, life-threatening heart rhythm problems, death, and permanent disability. Please reconsider. If you insist on leaving, please remember that you can return to the ED at any time if you change your mind about admission, if your symptoms change or worsen, or if other problems arise. Take four 81-mg baby aspirin every morning in addition to your other prescribed medications. Call both your family doctor and your cardiologist first thing in the morning to schedule appointments within 24 hours."

Accessing/Editing the Chart After a Bad Outcome

There will be situations when a provider is informed after a patient is discharged that a bad outcome has occurred. Providers will often review their charting in this situation and may be tempted to change their documentation. One of the most common pieces of advice given by malpractice defense attorneys is to avoid this temptation. It is almost always counterproductive.

EMRs detect and record when a chart is accessed and any changes that were made. The term "metadata" is defined as "descriptive data that characterizes other data to create a clearer understanding of their meaning and to achieve greater reliability and quality of information."[18] The Sedona Conference glossary adds "Metadata can describe how, when and by whom ESI (electronically stored information) was collected, created, accessed, modified and how it is formatted. [Metadata] [c]an be altered intentionally or inadvertently. Certain metadata can be extracted when native files are processed for litigation."[19] The American College of Emergency Physicians refers to metadata as a "treasure trove of information for plaintiff attorneys."[20] Although state laws vary,[21] metadata is discoverable in civil trials by federal law[22] and can be used to verify the timing and content of changes made to the medical record.

CONTROVERSIES/PITFALLS
Timing of Documentation

Although it can be difficult in a busy ED, we recommend that documentation be completed in real time whenever possible. This is especially important for the history and physical examination, as this allows for more accurate recollection of details. It is also helpful for consultants to have access to this information during patient encounters. The timing of MDM documentation is more controversial. Documenting this section of the chart in real time allows for accurate documentation of timing of events, including procedures, consultations, and test results. Providers who delay MDM documentation until the end of the patient encounter have the potential benefit of having hindsight when documenting their encounter, which may decrease malpractice risk and provide a "hard stop" for evaluating their own decision making regarding diagnosis, treatment, and disposition, as discussed above. When not able to document in real time, we recommend prioritizing documenting objective elements, including interventions, testing results, and consultations especially in critically ill patients in real time while documenting subjective decision making, such as disposition and diagnoses, at the end of the encounter.

Differential Diagnosis

Differential diagnosis formulation is a fundamental tool used in Emergency Medicine. Although developing and working through a differential diagnosis is universal, there is controversy surrounding how to or even whether to document this in the chart. Documenting a differential diagnosis may provide the benefit of explaining a provider's thought process when evaluating a patient. However, there are many potential pitfalls, such as listing a diagnosis in the differential that is not adequately tested for or ruled out, or documenting a list of potential diagnoses that does not include the eventual diagnosis. It is important that the provider explains why a diagnosis in the differential is unlikely with some combination of history and examination findings, testing results, decision-making tools, and other objective data. This is even more important if the diagnosis is one that is life threatening or requires an emergent intervention. We recommend documenting the rationale for ruling in or out any diagnosis listed in the differential, especially if associated with high morbidity and mortality. We discourage using standardized differential diagnosis lists for specific chief complaints, such as chest pain or shortness of breath, for the reasons noted above. If a differential is documented, each listed potential diagnosis should be adequately addressed, and we recommend including a statement that the diagnoses considered included but were not limited to those listed.

Templates

Templates allow for efficiency and faster documentation. They also provide potential pitfalls and risk, as they can lead to inaccurate documentation. Examples include documenting normal pedal pulses in a patient with a lower extremity amputation or documenting normal speech and mental status in a nonverbal or demented patient. If using templates for physical examination findings, we recommend creating a personal template that accurately incorporates examination elements that you consistently perform. This will help prevent documentation of findings that were not tested or evaluated, which will prevent inaccuracies or fraudulent medical billing.

Knowing exactly what is in the template or templates being used is important to assure that the template is edited for abnormal findings, for examination elements in the template that were not performed, and for more detailed examination elements that were performed that are not in the template. Templates should not be used in the HPI or MDM, as these sections are difficult to standardize and should be unique to each patient encounter. Inaccuracies can be used by plaintiff attorneys to suggest a provider is untruthful or sloppy and could threaten the provider's credibility with a jury.

In summary, templates should be used cautiously, reviewed for accuracy as they pertain to the specific patient encounter, should only include findings that are routinely evaluated for in all patients with similar presentations, and should periodically be reviewed and updated for changes in the provider's standard practice.

Point-of-Care Ultrasound

Emergency providers should perform and document point-of-care ultrasounds that are used to answer focused clinical questions.[23] It is necessary to document the following elements for both billing and medicolegal purposes: medical indication, body location scanned, interpretation, and images obtained and stored.[24] From a medicolegal perspective as well as from the perspective of consultants viewing the scans, including multiple images provides more information and better context. A clear image and correct interpretation are medicolegally protective; conversely, an unclear image that does not support the interpretation or a clear image that is not consistent with the interpretation could be medicolegally damaging.

Sign Out

The process of patient turnover between emergency providers is fraught with medicolegal danger. In fact, the American College of Emergency Physicians has identified it as one of the most dangerous procedures performed in the ED.[20] Transfers of care should be documented in the initial providers note, including time of transfer of care, important clinical information discussed, and agreement of the provider accepting the patient.[25] If an Emergency provider receives a sign out on a patient before they are dispositioned, the provider should document a brief HPI and document any new test results, changes in clinical status, treatments or interventions, and disposition decision in real time. This provides a continuation in MDM and justification for management, as well as providing consultants' complete and accurate information on a patient's course. At the end of shift, it is best to complete notes on all patients, but particularly on active patients before signing out. This provides the oncoming provider with useful clinical information to use as a reference, especially if there is an unexpected diagnostic test result or change in clinical status.

SUMMARY

Most emergency physicians will be named in a lawsuit at some point during their careers. When a case is brought to trial, the chart will be the primary source of information, not the faded memories of a long past patient encounter. The clinician's focus should be on the purposes of documentation (communication with other medical professionals, billing and coding, and medicolegal documentation) and developing techniques to summarize and tell the story of the encounter as seen through their eyes.

This approach will decrease the chance a lawsuit gets filed, and that if it does, that it will end with a plaintiff decision.

CLINICS CARE POINTS

- To the extent possible, complete charts in real time in order to most accurately reflect the encounter. Complete the History of Present Illness and Medical Decision Making at the time of service.

- Use the MDM as a "hard stop" to assure that the clinical decisions made during the course of the patient's care are justified by the charting, and any additional information or intervention can be performed while the patient is still in the department.

- Proper application and documentation of the concepts of decision-making capacity, shared decision making, informed refusal, informed consent and against medical advice are important not only to good patient care but also to a legally defensible chart.

- Avoid the pitfalls of electronic medical records checkboxes and templates by checking for accuracy and providing free text edits to assure that the chart tells the story of the patient encounter as the provider saw it.

- Recognize the danger of patient sign outs and handoffs from both patient care and medicolegal perspectives. Implement a standard procedure for these scenarios, and document them in the chart.

- Avoid the temptation to make additions or edits to the chart when there is a bad outcome or when a legal action is filed.

DISCLOSURE

The authors have nothing to disclose.

REFERENCES

1. Pallaci M, Markowski K, Weinstock M, Adler J. Emergency medicine documentation (US). In: Whitney J, Nordt S, Mattu A, Swadron S, editors. CorePendium. Burbank, CA: LLC; 2023. Available at: https://www.emrap.org/corependium/chapter/recXKF8nep5mkJcl3/Emergency-Medicine-Documentation-US#h.psmi9sbv7xtl. [Accessed 2 February 2024].
2. Jena AB, Seabury S, Lakdawalla D, et al. Malpractice risk according to physician specialty. N Engl J Med 2011;365(7):629–36.
3. Studdert DM, Mello MM, Sage WM, et al. Defensive medicine among high-risk specialist physicians in a volatile malpractice environment. J Am Med Assoc 2005;293(21):2609–17.
4. Reschovsky JD, Saiontz-Martinez CB. Malpractice claim fears and the costs of treating medicare patients: a new approach to estimating the costs of defensive medicine. Health Serv Res 2018;53(3):1498–516.
5. Hickson GB, Federspiel CF, Pichert JW, et al. Patient complaints and malpractice risk. JAMA 2002;287(22):2951–7.
6. Levinson W, Roter DL, Mullooly JP, et al. Physician-patient communication: the relationship with malpractice claims among primary care physicians and surgeons. J Am Med Assoc 1997;277(7):553–9.
7. Kellermann AL, Jones SS. What it will take to achieve the as-yet-unfulfilled promises of health information technology. Health Aff 2013;32(1):63–8.

8. Friedberg MW, Chen PG, Van Busum KR, et al. Factors affecting physician professional satisfaction and their implications for patient care, Health systems, and health policy, RAND Corporation, RR-439-AMA. 2013. Available at: https://www.rand.org/pubs/research_reports/RR439.html. [Accessed 30 January 2024].

9. Poissant L, Pereira J, Tamblyn R, et al. The impact of electronic health records on time efficiency of physicians and nurses: a systematic review. J Am Med Inform Assoc 2005;12(5):505–16.

10. Hill RG Jr, Sears LM, Melanson SW. 4000 clicks: a productivity analysis of electronic medical records in a community hospital ED. Am J Emerg Med 2013; 31(11):1591–4.

11. Mangalmurti SS, Murtagh L, Mello MM. Medical malpractice liability in the age of electronic health records. N Engl J Med 2010;363(21):2060–7.

12. Kuhn T, Basch P, Barr M, et al, Medical Informatics Committee of the American College of Physicians. Clinical documentation in the 21st century: executive summary of a policy position paper from the American College of Physicians. Ann Intern Med 2015;162(4):301–3.

13. AMA. CPT evaluation and management (E/M) code and guidelines changes. Chicago, IL: American Medical Association; 2022. Available at: https://www.ama-assn.org/system/files/2023-e-m-descriptors-guidelines.pdf.

14. Walker K, Ben-Meir M, Dunlop W, et al. Impact of scribes on emergency medicine doctors' productivity and patient throughput: multicentre randomised trial. BMJ 2019;364:l121.

15. The Joint Commission. Informed consent: more than getting a signature. Quick safety: an advisory on safety & quality issues. Oak Brook, IL: Joint Commission Resources; 2016. p. 4–5.

16. Palmer BW, Harmell AL. Assessment of healthcare decision-making capacity. Arch Clin Neuropsychol 2016;31(6):530–40.

17. Hess EP, Grudzen CR, Thomson R, et al. Shared decision-making in the emergency department: respecting patient autonomy when seconds count. Acad Emerg Med 2015;22(7):856–64.

18. AHIMA. Rules for handling and maintaining metadata in the EHR. J AHIMA (Am Health Inf Manag Assoc) 2013;84(5):50–4. Available at: https://library.ahima.org/doc?oid=106378#.YNOIki2caJ9. [Accessed 23 June 2021].

19. The sedona conference glossary: e-discovery & digital information management, 2010, Third Edition.

20. American College of Emergency Physicians. Top 10 principles on how to avoid getting sued in emergency medicine; an information paper developed by members of the ACEP medical legal committee. Available at: https://www.acep.org/globalassets/uploads/uploaded-files/acep/clinical-and-practice-management/resources/medical-legal/top-10-principles-on-how-to-avoid-getting-sued-in-em.pdf. [Accessed 1 February 2024].

21. Miller AR, Tucker CE. Electronic discovery and electronic medical records: does the threat of litigation affect firm decisions to adopt technology? Washington, DC: Federal Trade Commission; 2009. Available at: http://www.ftc.gov/be/seminardocs/090430amiller.pdf.

22. Lorenzetti DL, Quan H, Lucyk K, et al. Strategies for improving physician documentation in the emergency department: a systematic review. BMC Emerg Med 2018;18(1):36.

23. ACEP emergency ultrasound guidelines. Available at: https://www.acep.org/globalassets/new-pdfs/policy-statements/ultrasound-guidelines—emergency-point-of-care-and-clinical-ultrasound-guidelines-in-medicine.pdf.

24. Aziz S, Bottomley J, Mohandas V, et al. Improving the documentation quality of point-of-care ultrasound scans in the emergency department. BMJ Open Qual 2020;9(1):e000636.
25. Cheung DS, Kelly JJ, Beach C, et al, Section of Quality Improvement and Patient Safety, American College of Emergency Physicians. Improving handoffs in the emergency department. Ann Emerg Med 2010;55(2):171–80.

Pediatric High-Risk Conditions

Alyssa Kettler, MD[a,*], Ilene Claudius, MD[b,c]

KEYWORDS

- Malpractice • Appendicitis • Meningitis • Testicular torsion

KEY POINTS

- Cardiopulmonary arrest, meningitis, testicular torsion, and appendicitis are common sources of litigation in Pediatric Emergency Medicine.
- Delays in diagnosis are common causes of malpractice claims.
- Failure to perform a lumbar puncture or ultrasound is a common claim in malpractice cases.

INTRODUCTION TO PEDIATRIC MALPRACTICE LITIGATION

The ultimate goal when caring for children in the emergency department (ED) and urgent care is to differentiate those children who need urgent medical attention from those who do not. Practitioners encounter many obstacles including high volume, finite resources, variability of presentation, incomplete information, and other inherent limitations in our tests/workup. It is important to be aware of the common situations that result in suboptimal care that can translate to malpractice claims, morbidity, and even mortality.

A study by Glerum and colleagues in 2021 examined the composition of malpractice claims in the ED and urgent care settings from the years of 2001 to 2015, finding

1. Nine percent of pediatric malpractice claims involved care in US EDs or urgent care settings.
2. Patient death was reported in 31% of claims.
3. Regardless of underlying medical condition, 41% of cases claimed "error in diagnosis" as the chief medical factor leading to the claim.

[a] Pediatric Emergency Medicine, Department of Emergency Medicine, Harbor-UCLA Medical Center, Torrance, CA, USA; [b] Department of Emergency Medicine, Harbor-UCLA Medical Center, 1000 West Carson Street, N14, Torrance, CA 90509, USA; [c] Department of Emergency Medicine, UCLA, Los Angeles, CA, USA
* Corresponding author. Department of Emergency Medicine, 1000 West Carson Street, Torrance, CA 90502.
E-mail address: akettler@dhs.lacounty.gov

Emerg Med Clin N Am 43 (2025) 41–56
https://doi.org/10.1016/j.emc.2024.05.023
0733-8627/25/© 2024 Elsevier Inc. All rights are reserved, including those for text and data mining, AI training, and similar technologies.
emed.theclinics.com

4. The highest average compensation resulted from cases that failed to admit or delayed admission.
5. The most common disorders, in order of prevalence, were cardiorespiratory arrest, appendicitis, disorder of male genital organs, and encephalopathy/meningitis.

These conditions are similar in prevalence to the analysis conducted by Selbst and colleagues in 2005 that examined the composition of malpractice claims in ED and urgent care settings from the year 1985 to 2000. During these years, meningitis was more common than appendicitis, which was followed by upper extremity fractures and testicular torsion.[1] Meningitis, appendicitis, and testicular torsion remain common conditions involved in pediatric malpractices cases and deserve special consideration to prevent future adverse outcomes. Although the condition of cardiorespiratory arrest is cited as the most common reason for malpractice, this term represents a final common pathway of heterogeneous disorders. Therefore, this article will focus on specifics of meningitis, appendicitis, and testicular torsion, and the analysis of cardiorespiratory arrest will be deferred. However, it is important to acknowledge arrest as a common source of litigation and insure timely and thorough documentation.

MENINGITIS

Meningitis is typically broken into bacterial versus aseptic (which incorporates viral, fungal, protozoan/helminth, and even noninfectious causes such as autoimmune disorders, drug-induced, and oncologic processes).[2,3] Although individual situations vary, the most accepted definition of aseptic meningitis is cerebrospinal fluid (CSF) pleocytosis (white blood cell [WBC] count >5 cells/mm^3) with a negative Gram stain.[4] Less rigorous testing is performed on aseptic meningitis, particularly when it comes to suspected viral causes. The management of bacterial and viral meningitis is different and will be discussed in later section. Meningitis due to viral etiology is typically self-limited and does not have definitive/targeted treatment. For these reasons, a causative pathogen is only elucidated about 10% of the time.[3]

It is important to first divide pediatric groups by age since the causative organisms and presentations are not the same. Then meningitis should be characterized by etiology, as time course and management are different between the bacterial and aseptic (or nonbacterial) groups.

Neonatal Meningitis

Incidence/etiology
Some of the most vulnerable in our population are the neonates (age <28 days). In this age group, the primary mechanism of developing meningitis is bacteremia that spreads to the central nervous system (CNS); therefore, there may be concomitant sepsis at the time of meningitis diagnosis.[5] Between days of life 1 and 28, the most common cause of bacterial meningitis is Group B *Streptococcus* followed by *Escherichia coli*.[2] Cases of neonatal aseptic viral meningitis are typically caused by human parechovirus 3, a close relative to enterovirus and rhinovirus.[6]

Clinical presentation
The clinical signs/symptoms of neonatal meningitis overlap considerably with signs/symptoms of sepsis. Less than 2 months of age, the typical presentation of meningitis is irritability, abnormal sleep pattern, fever, vomiting, and decreased oral intake.[7] A unique symptom with low prevalence but potentially high specificity is paradoxic irritability, seen when the infant becomes more agitated with handling due to movement of the meninges.[8] These symptoms are unfortunately nonspecific and do not always

indicate a CNS infection. Presence of seizures and bulging fontanel may help indicate that the neonate has meningitis, but these are often late findings.[5,7,9]

Workup/management
No clinical prediction rules or constellation of serum tests are sufficient to exclude bacterial meningitis without performing a lumbar puncture (LP).[5] Among serum studies, C-reactive protein (CRP) and white blood cell (WBC) count do not perform well as screening tests for meningitis and should not be used to inform the decision to perform an LP. Procalcitonin has a sensitivity of 90% at detecting serious bacterial infection, but it does not help differentiate between septic neonates with and without meningitis. Blood cultures are negative in more than half of neonates with meningitis[2]; therefore, a negative blood culture is not a reason to defer an LP.

Baseline cellular levels in uninfected CSF vary based on age, particularly between the preterm and full-term neonate age groups. Typically, CSF WBC count and glucose levels are the same between preterm and full-term neonates; protein is significantly higher in the preterm population (209 vs 159 mg/dL, $P < .001$). This difference decreases as the infant ages.[10] A study by Garges and colleagues in 2005 examined noninfected CSF parameters (WBC, glucose, and protein) against CSF culture-proven bacterial meningitis in neonates ($\leq$34 week's gestation) but were unable to find a single parameter that could reliably rule in or rule out bacterial meningitis. Notably, 5% of the neonates with culture-proven bacterial meningitis in their study had either 0 or 1 CSF WBC per cubic millimeter and 20% had 3 or less CSF WBCs per cubic millimeter. CSF glucose and protein were highly variable and unreliable in terms of diagnosing bacterial meningitis.[11] To further complicate CSF interpretation, traumatic LPs are estimated to occur greater than 35% of the time in the neonatal population. Attempts to adjust for a pathologic WBC count based on the number of red cells in settings of traumatic taps have yielded a decrease in sensitivity with only marginal gains in specificity.[12]

Pediatric Meningitis

Incidence/etiology
In the modern vaccine era, there has been significant decline in cases of bacterial meningitis, but countries with high vaccination rates still report a bacterial cause in 3% to 18% of childhood meningitis cases.[2] In **Table 1**, the percentages of leading pathogens causing bacterial meningitis in fully vaccinated individuals are broken down by age grouping. Of viral causes, 95% of cases are due to enterovirus and human parechovirus. Other regularly identified viral causes include herpes simplex and varicella-zoster viruses.[2] Of note, meningoencephalitis from the latter 2 viruses bear substantial morbidity and mortality and require aggressive diagnosis and management.

Clinical presentation
The vast majority of providers are able to identify and treat the ill-appearing child with meningitis, but how can we keep from missing the child with the atypical presentation that is at-risk for decompensation? Amarilyo and colleagues in 2011 sought out to determine the specificity and sensitivity of presenting symptoms and physical examination findings (**Table 2**).[13] They enrolled 108 pediatric patients with symptoms concerning for meningitis (ages 2 months to 16 years old) from 2 EDs between February 1, 2006 and October 31, 2007 and diagnosed meningitis in 58 patients (53.7%) with 6 being bacterial and 52 being aseptic. By far the most sensitive finding was fever (93%), but it was very nonspecific. Conversely, Glasgow Coma Scale (GCS) less than 13 was very specific but not very sensitive. The authors identified that a child presenting with headache and positive Brudzinski and Kernig signs has the highest probability of

Table 1 Percentages of leading pathogens causing bacterial meningitis and viral meningitis in fully vaccinated individuals are broken down by age grouping		
	Pathogen Percentages in Meningitis	
Age Range	**Bacterial Meningitis**	**Viral Meningitis**
<1 mo	Group B *Streptococcus* (30%) and *E coli* (30%)	Nonpolio enterovirus* (80%– 95%), human parechovirus, herpes simplex, and varicella-zoster
1 to <3 mo	Group B *Streptococcus* (39%) and Gram-negative rods (32%)	
≥3 mo to <10 y	*Streptococcus pneumococcus* (45%–47%) and *Neisseria meningitidis* (32%–34%)	
10+ y	*N meningitidis* (55%) and *S pneumococcus* (21%)	

*Nonpolio Enteroviruses include coxsackieviruses A and B, echoviruses, the newer numbered enteroviruses 68 to 71.[59]

Information in the following table was extrapolated from Mijovic and colleagues 2019, Nigrovic and colleagues 2008, Xu and colleagues 2019, Hviid and colleagues 2007, and Sawyer 2001. [2,56,59–61]

meningitis (positive predictive value [PPV] 87.5%). Unfortunately, only a few patients in their entire study fit this constellation of signs/symptoms.

Workup/management

If meningitis is on the differential, an LP and analysis of the CSF should occur as quickly as feasibly and safely as possible.

As opposed to the neonatal age group, there are CSF value-based prediction rules designed for children aged 29 days and older with CSF pleocytosis. The goal of these scoring tests, The Bacterial Meningitis Score (BMS) and Meningitest, are to assist with identifying children who are at low risk of bacterial meningitis, despite having pleocytosis in their CSF.[2,14] A meta-analysis of BMS yields a sensitivity of 99.3% and a negative predictive value (NPV) of 99.7%.[14] BMS has been more rigorously validated with a larger number of patients than Meningitest; therefore, we will discuss BMS components in the next section.[14,15] Of note, neither clinical decision rule (CDR) can be applied to children with history of neurosurgical intervention, immunosuppression, pretreatment with antibiotics, traumatic spinal tap, and septic shock.[14,15]

Understanding the properties of CSF and how they change with treatment is important to its analysis. With administration of intravenous antibiotics, CSF sterility can be achieved in 15 minutes to 2 hours with *N meningitidis*, 4 to 6 hours with *S pneumoniae*, and 8 hours with Group B *Streptococcus*.[16,17] CSF WBC start to degrade within 90 minutes.[17,18] These are short time windows in which to obtain CSF for a chance of positive culture and/or accurate CSF fluid components. Luckily in today's modern era of nucleic acid amplification tests (such as polymerase chain reaction [PCR]), the requirement of viable bacteria in CSF is no longer mandatory. In fact, multiple studies have found that PCR is more sensitive than the longtime gold standard of CSF culture in identification of pathogens.[19–21] Despite these advances in technology, it is important to note that in approximately 40% of cases where children are admitted for suspected bacterial meningitis, no causative pathogen is ever identified.[2]

Differentiating aseptic from bacterial meningitis in the pediatric population/clinical decision rule

All meningitis is not created equal. Aseptic (aka nonbacterial) meningitis accounts for the vast majority of the cases of meningitis in the modern vaccine era. The clinical

Table 2
Presenting symptoms and signs of the study groups on admission (n = 108)

	No. Patients[a]	Meningitis[b] Sensitivity, %	95% Confidence Interval Sensitivity	Meningitis[c]	Specificity	95% Confidence Interval Specificity	PPV	Odds Ratio	95% Confidence Interval	P
Headaches	61 (56%)	32[d]/42 (76%)	0.6–0.86	9[e]/19 (47%)	0.53	0.29–0.74	0.78	3.5	1.1–11.1	.026
Vomiting, nausea	108 (100%)	41/58 (71%)	0.57–0.81	19/50 (38%)	0.62	0.47–0.75	0.68	4.1	1.8–9.4	.01
Photophobia	69 (64%)	12/43 (28%)	0.16–0.44	3/26 (12%)	0.88	0.69–0.97	0.8	2.9	0.75–11.7	.11
Motor deficiency	108 (100%)	2/58 (3%)	0–0.13	1/50 (2%)	0.98	0.88–0.99	0.67	1.7	0.14–19	.67
Seizures	108 (100%)	11/58 (19%)	0.1–0.32	18/50 (36%)	0.64	0.49–0.77	0.38	0.37	0.15–0.9	.028
Fever[f]	108 (100%)	54[d]/58 (93%)	0.82–0.98	46[e]/50 (92%)	0.08	0.02–0.2	0.54	1.1	0.22–6	.86
GCS <13	108 (100%)	5/58 (9%)	0.03–0.2	4/50 (8%)	0.92	0.8–0.97	0.56	1.05	0.26–4.1	.94
Nuchal rigidity	79 (73%)	32/49 (65%)	0.5–0.77	10/30 (33%)	0.67	0.47–0.82	0.8	4.8	2–11.4	.01
Brudzinski sign	79 (73%)	25/49 (51%)	0.36–0.65	6/30 (20%)	0.8	0.63–0.92	0.81	4.3	1.5–12.3	.004
Kernig sign	79 (73%)	13/49 (27%)	0.15–0.41	4/30 (13%)	0.87	0.68–0.96	0.77	2.3	0.66–7.8	.19
Bulging fontanel	31 (29%)	5/10 (50%)	0.2–0.8	8/21 (38%)	0.62	0.39–0.81	0.38	0.6	0.13–2.8	.54

[a] Patients for whom all required data were available.
[b] Final diagnosis of meningitis.
[c] Final diagnosis not meningitis.
[d] Number of patients with a positive sign in the meningitis group.
[e] Number of patients with a positive sign in the nonmeningitis group.
[f] Fever was defined as rectal temperature higher than 38°C.

Amarilyo G, Alper A, Ben-Tov A, Grisaru-Soen G. Diagnostic accuracy of clinical symptoms and signs in children with meningitis. Pediatr Emerg Care. 2011 Mar;27(3):196-9.

course for aseptic meningitis is typically one of a self-limited condition that needs only supportive care. In contrast, bacterial meningitis carries the risk of high morbidity and mortality. As discussed earlier, there is no single value from CSF that is able to reliably rule in or rule out bacterial meningitis. Utilizing the BMS can help to effectively rule out bacterial meningitis in patients aged 29 days to 19 years with CSF WBC count of 10 cells/µL or greater. If a patient does *not* have any of the following parameters, then there is a very low risk of bacterial meningitis with an NPV of 99.7%.[14]

1. Positive Gram stain
2. CSF absolute neutrophile count (ANC) 1000 cells/µL or greater
3. CSF protein 80 g/dL or greater (800 mg/L)
4. Peripheral blood ANC 10,000 cells/µL or greater
5. Seizure at (or prior to) initial presentation

Meningoencephalitis

Infections of the CNS are on a spectrum, depending on which structures are infected/ inflamed. Overall, meningitis is a much more common occurrence compared to encephalitis. Clinically, when cerebral function becomes compromised, such as altered behavior, motor dysfunction, or speech impairment, the condition would be classified as encephalitis rather than meningitis. Because patients can have meningitis, encephalitis, or meningoencephalitis, clinical features vary. Isolated encephalitis often presents without classic nuchal rigidity, which can discourage the clinician from pursuing a diagnosis of an intracranial infection and lead to important diagnostic error. Of the infectious causes of encephalitis, herpes simplex virus is the most common, which is typically acquired perinatally.

Time Course of Meningococcal (N meningitidis) Meningitis

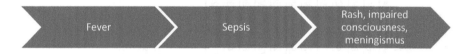

Thompson and colleagues found most children displayed nonspecific symptoms in the first 4 to 6 hours followed by rapid progression to near mortality within 24 hours. The first symptom described by children (or their parents) was fever in ages less than 5 years old and headache in ages greater than 5 years old.[22] The difficulty is that symptoms are nonspecific and are often due to self-limiting illness. In all age groups, signs of sepsis (abnormal skin color, cold hands/feet) were the next to develop. In the younger age group, drowsiness and rapid/labored breathing were also noted. The first classic/specific sign to suggest meningococcemia is rash, but this does not develop till after signs of sepsis are present and often starts as a nonspecific rash, turning into the petechial/hemorrhagic form over the course of hours.[22] Notably, the classic meningeal signs of neck stiffness, photophobia, and bulging fontanelle did not present till well into the disease course, 12 to 15 hours after onset of symptoms. The late findings such as unconsciousness and seizure did not develop until about 15 hours in infants and 24 hours in older children.[22]

When to computed tomography before lumbar puncture?

A feared complication of LP is that removal of spinal fluid in a patient with elevated intracranial pressure (such as a space occupying lesion) can cause a relative pressure gradient and precipitate brainstem herniation, leading to significant neurologic morbidity and/or mortality.[23] The exact incidence of this complication is unknown but the range is believed to be between 0.1% and 3%, likely closer to 0.1%.[24] Although no formal criteria exist on when to get a head computed tomography (CT) prior to LP in the pediatric population, recommendations can be extrapolated from the adult population, which include

- Altered mental status
- Focal neurologic deficit
- New-onset seizure
- Papilledema
- Historical risk factors (immunocompromised state, malignancy, history of focal CNS disease, and concern for mass CNS lesion).[25]

Costerus and colleagues in 2017 conducted a study of herniation risk after LP in the setting of bacterial meningitis. In the study, 1533 cases of community-acquired bacterial meningitis in patients aged greater than 16 years were included. Forty-seven (3.1%) of those patients had clinical deterioration within 8 hours of their LP. Forty-three out of 47 had CT scans performed before the LP. Seventeen (40%) were read as normal and 13 (30%) were read as generalized edema. The remaining reads included hydrocephalus, intracranial air, metastasis, old vascular abnormalities, and focal edema.[24]

Twenty-two of the 47 cases of clinical deterioration had a repeat head CT and 10 (45%) showed cerebral herniation.[24] However, it is unclear if the rate of herniation is due to the bacterial meningitis, the LP, or a combination of the two. Ultimately, it is important to perform a screening head CT on those who meet high risk criteria, but LPs are well tolerated procedures with low complication rates (**Fig. 1**).

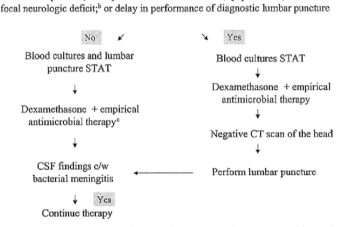

Fig. 1. Practice guideline in pediatric bacterial meningitis (age >1 month). [a]Includes those with CSF shunts, hydrocephalus, trauma, status-post neurosurgery, or space-occupying lesion; [b]Palsy of cranial nerve VI or VII is not an indication to delay lumbar puncture; [c]Dexamethasone and antimicrobial therapy should be administered immediately after CSF is obtained.[23] (Tunkel AR, Hartman BJ, Kaplan SL, et al. Practice Guidelines for the Management of Bacterial Meningitis. Clinical Infectious Diseases. 2004 Nov 1; 39(9): 1267–1284.)

Techniques to Decrease Medicolegal Risk

Where do providers go wrong in their treatment of meningitis? What can we learn from malpractice cases of the past? Examination of data from the Physician Insurers Association of America (PIAA) Meningitis Claims study found the following statistics:[26]

1. Sixty percent of claims involved patients aged less than 2 years.
2. Of the cases that involved patient death, 82.6% were aged less than 1 year.
3. The most common malpractice cited in these cases was delay in diagnosis.
4. In 57.5% of cases, treatment was sought within 24 hours of symptom onset.
5. Antibiotics were given within 24 hours of initial medical contact in only 49% of cases.
6. Only 30% of patients presented to the ED as their first point of medical contact.
7. In a quarter of cases of missed meningitis, patients had no fever.
8. The majority of patients with missed meningitis lacked mental status changes, headache, lethargy, and neck stiffness.
9. In almost 30% of cases, no LP was performed.

Given the only vague presentation involved in missed cases of meningitis, the clinician must maintain an incredibly high index of suspicion for meningitis, especially in the neonates/infants. In addition to management claims of malpractice, McAbee and colleagues found that 12% of PIAA meningitis claims noted grievances in regards to medical charting. Additionally, communication issues were cited as impacting delay in diagnosis. These areas of breakdown are listed as follows:

1. Failure to document standards of practice
2. Failure to record pertinent negative findings
3. Failure to document interactions with the patient/family
4. Failure to record referrals consults/referrals to other physicians
5. Poor communication between providers
6. Failure to inform patient/family of critical test results
7. Failure to provide consultants with complete medical findings/history
8. Lack of clear follow-up instructions[26]

Take home points/techniques to decrease medicolegal risk

1. Have a high index of suspicion for bacterial meningitis in children aged less than 2 years, especially because symptoms can be subtle.
2. Err on the side of getting the LP.
3. There are no constellation of signs/symptoms with high enough negative predictive value to rule out bacterial meningitis. Lack of fever does not exclude meningitis.
4. Give antibiotics early, especially if you anticipate any delays due to obtaining a head CT or performing an LP.
5. Meningococcemia can progress rapidly. A period of several hours of observation can often assist with decision-making regarding LP.

APPENDICITIS
Introduction/Pathophysiology

Appendicitis is an inflammation of the appendix, most commonly caused by the obstruction of the lumen by an appendicolith or foreign body, lymphoid hyperplasia, parasites, or tumor burden.[27] A common disease involved in malpractice cases, this condition has variable presentation and carries significant morbidity and mortality. There are multiple factors that make diagnosing appendicitis difficult including limited history due to patient age, lack of cooperation during physical examination, difficulty balancing throughput and observation, desire to limit ionizing radiation, and inferior sensitivity/specificity of scoring systems. In order to improve patient outcomes and reduce legal risk, clinicians need to be knowledgeable about the common causes of malpractice cases, which elements of the history and physical are useful in diagnosis, and the predictive value of CDRs/laboratory tests/imaging.

Clinical Presentation/History/Physical examination

The first step in evaluating a pediatric patient for appendicitis is history and physical, though appendicitis is notorious for having a variable presentation. Textbooks commonly teach that the pain should start in the umbilical region and then migrate to the right lower quadrant, but this classic presentation is present in the minority of cases.[28] A systematic review of 21 studies by Benabbas and colleagues in 2017 showed the following historical elements and physical examination findings that increase likelihood of appendicitis.

1. "Pain migration to right lower quadrant" had a positive likelihood ratio of only 1.75
2. In a single study by Goldman and colleagues, the presence of "cough/hop pain" on physical examination in undifferentiated abdominal pain had a positive likelihood ratio of 7.64
3. Rovsing's sign on physical examination had a positive likelihood ratio of 3.52 but only a negative likelihood ratio of 0.72 in absence of the sign[29]

Although the aforementioned symptoms/physical examination findings increase the likelihood of having appendicitis, no finding alone was sufficient enough to rule in or rule out appendicitis.[29]

Clinical Decision Rules in Appendicitis

CDRs were developed as a tool to help providers make diagnostic and therapeutic decisions in a data-driven way. A systematic review conducted by Kulik and colleagues in 2013 examined the 2 most well-validated clinical prediction rules at the time, the pediatric appendicitis score (PAS) and the Alvarado score,[30] finding that while PAS outperformed Alvarado, neither CDR met performance benchmarks needed to be used in routine practice. An additional systematic review by Benabbas and colleagues in 2017[29] showed that a PAS score of 9 or greater had a positive likelihood ratio of 5.26 but none of the elements in the history, physical examination, laboratory findings, or PAS score could accurately rule in or rule out appendicitis. Specifically, 60% to 70% of patients were classified with a PAS score between 3 and 6, putting them in the equivocal group and yielding minimal aid to the diagnostician.[31–34] A new CDR was developed in 2018 called the pediatric appendicitis risk calculator (pARC) that outperformed PAS. Half of patients are classified into the low-risk or high-risk groups using pARC whereas only 23% of patients are classified as PAS less than 3 or greater than 8.[34] If the patient falls into the low-risk group, they can be safely discharged from the ED without advanced imaging. Conversely, patients in the high-risk category have sufficient pretest probability of appendicitis to forgo imaging and immediately consult pediatric surgery consultation. This obviates imaging in half of children.[34] The pARC provides the most utility in patients who would have been considered equivocal by the PAS.

Ultrasound in Appendicitis

A study by Cohen and colleagues in 2015 examined all pediatric ultrasounds that were obtained between 2004 and 2013 for evaluation for appendicitis (1383 in total). Of the

876 (63%) which were nondiagnostic, 777 scans (56%) had nonvisualization of the appendix. Based on their analysis, the negative predictive value of a negative ultrasound was 98.68%, which was consistent with previous studies. The negative predictive value of a nonvisualized appendix in a nondiagnostic study was only 86.36%. Authors also examined these variables to see how they impacted the negative predictive value in nonvisualized, nondiagnostic ultrasound studies to evaluate for appendicitis.

1. WBC less than 7.5×10^9/L increased the NPV to 98.86%
2. WBC less than 11.0×10^9/L increased the NPV to 96.99%
3. Age less than 5 years increased NPV to 91.40%
4. Female sex increased NPV to 88.72%[35]

With the ubiquitous use of ultrasound, it has become commonplace for a provider to interpret one that is nondiagnostic. There are a number of options, including supplementing with additional information, such as the WBC, additional imaging, serial examinations, a 12 to 24 hour recheck or a surgical consultation. Use of shared decision-making and documented communication to the family of diagnostic equipoise is paramount.

Computed Tomographic Scan to Evaluate for Appendicitis

A systematic review of 22 studies by Kim and colleagues in 2018 showed CT imaging for the evaluation of appendicitis in the pediatric population to have pooled sensitivity of 95% and pooled specificity of 94%. They also noted similar sensitivity and specificity in noncontrasted and low-dose radiation forms of CT imaging. Of patients with equivocal CT finding of appendicitis, 17% had appendicitis.[36]

Techniques to Decrease Medicolegal Risk

Where have previous providers gone wrong in their evaluation/management of pediatric appendicitis? Sullins and colleagues examined pediatric appendicitis malpractice claims between 1984 and 2013, identifying 158 cases for analysis. Key features include

- Seventy-four percent of cases claimed delay or failure in diagnosis of appendicitis.
- Within the group of delay or failure to diagnose, 62.9% of cases resulted in perforation, 24.5% suffered postoperative complications, and 19.9% resulted in death of patient.
- Half of the 158 cases went to trial and 68.4% of those cases sided in favor of the defense (medical practitioner).

Risk factors for misdiagnosis

What clinical situations are more likely to lead to diagnostic error? Mahajan and colleagues 2020 analyzed data from 22,336 children who had an ED visit within 30 days for a related symptom prior to being diagnosed with appendicitis and compared to children who were diagnosed with appendicitis at their initial visit. There were a total of 973 children in the potentially missed appendicitis group, accounting for approximately 4.4% of group analyzed. Authors also found statistically significant differences in demographics/composition of the potentially missed appendicitis group.

1. More likely to be female ($P < .001$)
2. More likely to have 2+ comorbidities ($P < .001$)
3. Lack of reported abdominal pain ($P < .001$, adjusted odds ratio [aOR] 2.99)
4. Concurrent abdominal pain and constipation ($P < .001$, aOR 2.43)[37]

Risk factors for perforation in appendicitis

Timely diagnosis is important in appendicitis due to the risk of perforation with diagnostic delays and subsequent morbidity and mortality.[38] Nelson and colleagues in 2000 sought to identify factors that correlate with a higher risk of perforation in appendicitis at the time of diagnosis. These authors identified the following statistically significant factors that increased the risk of perforation in appendicitis.

1. Younger age (8 year old [perforated appendicitis] vs 11 year old [unperforated appendicitis])
2. Longer duration of symptoms (3 days vs 1.4 days)
3. Presence of vomiting in the history of present illness (91% vs 69%)
4. Presence of fever in the history of present illness (83% vs 58%)
5. Higher median temperatures (39.0°C vs 38.3°C)
6. Higher proportions of leukocyte (WBC) bands (14% vs 5%)[38]

Additionally, a study by Michelson and colleagues in 2023 examined cases of missed appendicitis at 5 large children's hospitals in the United States. Of 30,702 cases of pediatric appendicitis, 429 were initially missed (1.39% miss rate). Adverse outcomes between the missed and discovered diagnosis groups found that the rate of abdominal abscess drainage was higher in the missed diagnosis group (13.5% compared to 4.7%, aOR 2.9, P <.001) and perforation rate was higher in the missed diagnosis group (64.3% compared to 33.5%, aOR 3.1, P <.001).[39]

Take home points/techniques to decrease medicolegal risk
- Most malpractice cases of appendicitis are due to missed or delayed diagnosis
- Risk factors for missed diagnosis include female sex, multiple comorbidities, and lack of abdominal pain
- Be particularly careful in children with concurrent abdominal pain and constipation
- As with many conditions, be particularly vigilant in children aged 3 years and under

TESTICULAR TORSION
Pathophysiology/Incidence

Testicular torsion is a time-sensitive medical emergency that develops when there is twisting of the spermatic cord and its contents. The most common age group affected is adolescent male individuals followed by smaller peak in the perinatal age group.[40] Risk factors for perinatal torsion include breech presentation, traumatic delivery, spasms/contraction of cremasteric muscles, and adduction contractures of the hips knowns as "scissor-leg deformity."[41,42] Conversely in the adolescent male group, testicular torsion is often caused by a congenital bell-clapper deformity, which is classically bilateral. Postsurgical loss of testicle is 34% to 42%.[43] Therefore, prompt surgical intervention is key. After 6 to 8 hours of symptoms in complete torsion with lack of arterial flow, the ability to salvage the testicle decreases.[40] This time range may be longer in cases of incomplete torsion/partial arterial flow. After detorsion and orchiopexy, the salvageable testes will undergo atrophy in 25% of cases due to the prolonged ischemia.[44]

Clinical Presentation

Two large-volume studies showed the incidence of testicular torsion in pediatric male individuals presenting to the ED with acute scrotal pain to be 3.25% and 10.2%.[45,46]

The Beni-Israel and colleagues study found 4 signs/symptoms were associated with an increased likelihood of testicular torsion including

- Pain less than 24 hours
- Nausea/vomiting
- High-riding testicle
- Abnormal cremasteric reflex.[45]

Importantly, absence of these factors does not rule out torsion. Five out of the 17 patients who had testicular torsion had a normal cremasteric reflex *and* half of the patients did not have a high-riding testicle. All patients had at least 1 of the 4 clinical predictors, and the absence of all 4 signs/symptoms is a high negative predictor value.[45] A remarkable percentage (31%) of patients can present with reports of abdominal pain rather than testicular pain, so it is imperative to perform a genitourinary examination on male individuals with abdominal pain.[47]

Ultrasound

Ultrasound is the imaging modality of choice in the evaluation for testicular torsion looking for twisting of the spermatic cord and decreased/absent testicular perfusion. Combining data from 5 pediatric studies on ultrasound for the diagnosis of testicular torsion yielded high sensitivity and specificity, 90% and 97.3%, respectively.[46,48–52] Of note, it is possible to have normal or increased flow in testicular torsion, especially in the early stages when there is venous dilation and preserved arterial flow. Therefore, additional ultrasound findings of testicular torsion must be examined including looking for a "whirlpool sign" in the spermatic cord indicating torsion.[53]

Management

Testicular torsion can be diagnosed based on history and physical alone if there are enough classic factors present. In these scenarios, urology should be consulted for immediate surgical management, and confirmatory imaging should not delay the surgical intervention.[40] In situations where there are delays in completion of imaging or surgical intervention, there are still maneuvers that can be deployed. There are case reports where emergency medicine providers performed bedside power Doppler ultrasound to diagnose testicular torsion and expedite surgical intervention and salvage of the testicle.[54] Given that the utility of ultrasound is user dependent, the greatest utility for bedside ultrasound would be to expedite surgical intervention or manual detorsion rather than attempting to rule out the presence of testicular torsion. If there is uncertainty, formal ultrasound should be obtained. In the setting that surgical intervention may be delayed, manual detorsion should be attempted. Described in the textbook *Fleisher & Ludwig*'s *Textbook of Pediatric Emergency Medicine*, the procedure should be preceded by adequate analgesia, and the procedure should be guided by the use of a bedside Doppler to hear if arterial flow returns. Approximately two-thirds of the time the torsion occurs medially, so the affected testicle should be rotated outward toward the thigh (medial to lateral, referred to as "opening the book"). More than one full 360° rotation may be needed. Successful detorsion should be marked by relief of pain, lower position of the testicle in the scrotum, and return of audible arterial flow with Doppler.[7] Manual detorsion does not obviate surgical intervention, since many causes continue to have partial torsion and/or are a risk for retorsion.[40] A study of routine manual detorsion in a pediatric ED showed an 80.5% success rate, and all manually detorsed testicles were perfused/viable at time of delayed surgical exploration and bilateral orchiopexy.[55]

Malpractice Data

Testicular torsion is a time-sensitive urologic emergency with significant consequences if missed, making it a classic set up for malpractice cases. Colaco and colleagues examine malpractice claims between the years 1990 and 2013. They included 52 cases in their analysis, 53% were minors. Key findings include:

- The majority of negligence claims were of failure to diagnose (96%).
- In cases pertaining to failure to diagnose, 72% of the time ultrasound was not used in the evaluation of the acute scrotal pain.
- Sixty-five percent of misdiagnosed cases were given an initial diagnosis of epididymitis.[57]

These findings stress the importance of performing ultrasound with complaints of testicular pain. Additionally, since testicular torsion is time sensitive, it is important to triage appropriately to reduce waiting time. There were a handful of cases that claimed delay in diagnosis due to prolonged wait times.[58] This is an easily avoidable issue, and triage protocols should be adjusted accordingly.

Take home points/techniques to decrease medicolegal risk

- After 6 to 8 hours of complete torsion, the rate of testicular salvage declines.
- Perform a genitourinary examination on all male individuals complaining of abdominal pain.
- Expeditious triage and early use of ultrasound can prevent delays in diagnosis/ treatment.
- If torsion is likely and they are any anticipated delays, manual detorsion should be attempted.

CLINICS CARE POINTS

- Meningitis can be subtle in early infancy.
- Delayed diagnosis of appendicitis can lead to perforation.
- Testicular torsion should be treated within 6 to 8 hours.

DISCLOSURE

The authors have nothing to disclose.

REFERENCES

1. Selbst SM, Friedman MJ, Singh SB. Epidemiology and etiology of malpractice lawsuits involving children in US emergency departments and urgent care centers. Pediatr Emerg Care 2005;21(3):165–9.
2. Mijovic H, Sadarangani M. To LP or not to LP? identifying the etiology of pediatric meningitis. Pediatr Infect Dis J 2019;38(6S Suppl 1):S39–42.
3. Kaur H, Betances EM, Perera TB. Aseptic meningitis. In: StatPearls [Internet]. Treasure Island (FL): StatPearls Publishing; 2024 [Updated 2022 May 29].
4. Tapiainen T, Prevots R, Izurieta HS, et al. Aseptic meningitis: case definition and guidelines for collection, analysis and presentation of immunization safety data. Vaccine 2007;25(31):5793–802.

5. Bedetti L, Marrozzini L, Baraldi A, et al. Pitfalls in the diagnosis of meningitis in neonates and young infants: the role of lumbar puncture. J Matern Fetal Neonatal Med 2019;32(23):4029–35.

6. Renaud C, Harrison CJ. Human parechovirus 3: the most common viral cause of meningoencephalitis in young infants. Infect Dis Clin 2015;29(3):415–28.

7. Shaw KN, Bachur RG. Chapter 31: fever. In: Florin TA, Cohn KA, Alpern ER, editors. Fleisher & Ludwig's textbook of pediatric emergency medicine. 8th edition. Philadelphia: Wolters Kluwer; 2021. p. 194–205.

8. Jones TW. Infectious meningitis: a focused review, Pediatr Emerg Med Rep, 23 (5)2018, 57-71.

9. Krebs VLJ, Costa GAM. Clinical outcome of neonatal bacterial meningitis according to birth weight. Arq Neuro Psiquiatr 2007;65(4b):1149–53.

10. Srinivasan L, Shah SS, Padula MA, et al. Cerebrospinal fluid reference ranges in term and preterm infants in the neonatal intensive care unit. J Pediatr 2012; 161(4):729–34.

11. Garges HP, Moody MA, Cotten CM, et al. Neonatal meningitis: what is the correlation among cerebrospinal fluid cultures, blood cultures, and cerebrospinal fluid parameters? Pediatrics 2006;117(4):1094–100.

12. Greenberg RG, Smith PB, Cotten CM, et al. Traumatic lumbar punctures in neonates: test performance of the cerebrospinal fluid white blood cell count. Pediatr Infect Dis J 2008;27(12):1047–51.

13. Amarilyo G, Alper A, Ben-Tov A, et al. Diagnostic accuracy of clinical symptoms and signs in children with meningitis. Pediatr Emerg Care 2011;27(3):196–9.

14. Nigrovic LE, Malley R, Kuppermann N. Meta-analysis of bacterial meningitis score validation studies. Arch Dis Child 2012;97(9):799–805.

15. Dubos F, Korczowski B, Aygun DA, et al. Distinguishing between bacterial and aseptic meningitis in children: European comparison of two clinical decision rules. Arch Dis Child 2010;95(12):963–7.

16. Riordan FA, Cant AJ. When to do a lumbar puncture. Arch Dis Child 2002;87(3): 235–7.

17. Kanegaye JT, Soliemanzadeh P, Bradley JS. Lumbar puncture in pediatric bacterial meningitis: defining the time interval for recovery of cerebrospinal fluid pathogens after parenteral antibiotic pretreatment. Pediatrics 2001;108(5):1169–74 [Erratum appears in Pediatrics 2002;110(3):651].

18. Connell T, Curtis N. How to interpret a CSF–the art and the science. Adv Exp Med Biol 2005;568:199–216.

19. Wu HM, Cordeiro SM, Harcourt BH, et al. Accuracy of real-time PCR, gram stain and culture for streptococcus pneumoniae, neisseria meningitidis and haemophilus influenzae meningitis diagnosis. BMC Infect Dis 2013;13:26.

20. Van Gastel E, Bruynseels P, Verstrepen W, et al. Evaluation of a real-time polymerase chain reaction assay for the diagnosis of pneumococcal and meningococcal meningitis in a tertiary care hospital. Eur J Clin Microbiol Infect Dis 2007;26(9):651–3.

21. Corless CE, Guiver M, Borrow R, et al. Simultaneous detection of neisseria meningitidis, haemophilus influenzae, and streptococcus pneumoniae in suspected cases of meningitis and septicemia using real-time PCR. J Clin Microbiol 2001; 39(4):1553–8.

22. Thompson MJ, Ninis N, Perera R, et al. Clinical recognition of meningococcal disease in children and adolescents. Lancet 2006;367(9508):397–403.

23. Tunkel AR, Hartman BJ, Kaplan SL, et al. Practice guidelines for the management of bacterial meningitis. Clin Infect Dis 2004;39(9):1267–84.

24. Costerus JM, Brouwer MC, Sprengers MES, et al. Cranial computed tomography, lumbar puncture, and clinical deterioration in bacterial meningitis: a nationwide cohort study. Clin Infect Dis 2018;67(6):920–6.
25. Tintinalli JE, Stapczynski JS, Ma OJ, et al. Chapter 174: central nervous system and spinal infections. In: Tanski ME, Ma OJ, editors. Tintinalli's emergency medicine. 8th edition. New York: McGraw Hill; 2016. p. 1192–9.
26. McAbee GN, Donn SM, Mendelson RA, et al. Medical diagnoses commonly associated with pediatric malpractice lawsuits in the United States. Pediatrics 2008; 122(6):e1282–6.
27. Howell EC, Dubina ED, Lee SL. Perforation risk in pediatric appendicitis: assessment and management. Pediatr Health Med Therapeut 2018;9:135–45.
28. Sullins VF, Rouch JD, Lee SL. Malpractice in cases of pediatric appendicitis. Clin Pediatr 2017;56(3):226–30.
29. Benabbas R, Hanna M, Shah J, et al. Diagnostic accuracy of history, physical examination, laboratory tests, and point-of-care ultrasound for pediatric acute appendicitis in the emergency department: a systematic review and meta-analysis. Acad Emerg Med 2017;24(5):523–51.
30. Kulik DM, Uleryk EM, Maguire JL. Does this child have appendicitis? a systematic review of clinical prediction rules for children with acute abdominal pain. J Clin Epidemiol 2013;66(1):95–104.
31. Schneider C, Kharbanda A, Bachur R. Evaluating appendicitis scoring systems using a prospective pediatric cohort. Ann Emerg Med 2007;49(6):778–84.
32. Bhatt M, Joseph L, Ducharme FM, et al. Prospective validation of the pediatric appendicitis score in a Canadian pediatric emergency department. Acad Emerg Med 2009;16(7):591–6.
33. Goldman RD, Carter S, Stephens D, et al. Prospective validation of the pediatric appendicitis score. J Pediatr 2008;153(2):278–82. Epub 2008 Mar 19. [Erratum appears in J Pediatr 2009;154(2):308–9].
34. Kharbanda AB, Vazquez-Benitez G, Ballard DW, et al. Development and validation of a novel pediatric appendicitis risk calculator (pARC). Pediatrics 2018; 141(4):e2017–699.
35. Cohen B, Bowling J, Midulla P, et al. The non-diagnostic ultrasound in appendicitis: is a non-visualized appendix the same as a negative study? J Pediatr Surg 2015;50(6):923–7.
36. Kim DW, Yoon HM, Lee JY, et al. Diagnostic performance of CT for pediatric patients with suspected appendicitis in various clinical settings: a systematic review and meta-analysis. Emerg Radiol 2018;25(6):627–37.
37. Mahajan P, Basu T, Pai C, et al. Factors associated with potentially missed diagnosis of appendicitis in the emergency department. JAMA Netw Open 2020;3(3): e200612.
38. Nelson DS, Bateman B, Bolte RG. Appendiceal perforation in children diagnosed in a pediatric emergency department. Pediatr Emerg Care 2000;16(4):233–7.
39. Michelson KA, Bachur RG, Grubenhoff JA, et al. Outcomes of missed diagnosis of pediatric appendicitis, new-onset diabetic ketoacidosis, and sepsis in five pediatric hospitals. J Emerg Med 2023;65(1):e9–18.
40. Bowlin PR, Gatti JM, Murphy JP. Pediatric testicular torsion. Surg Clin North Am 2017;97(1):161–72.
41. Riaz-Ul-Haq M, Mahdi DE, Elhassan EU. Neonatal testicular torsion; a review article. Iran J Pediatr 2012;22(3):281–9.
42. Naouar S, Braiek S, El Kamel R. Testicular torsion in undescended testis: a persistent challenge. Asian J Urol 2017;4(2):111–5.

43. Taghavi K, Dumble C, Hutson JM, et al. The bell-clapper deformity of the testis: The definitive pathological anatomy. J Pediatr Surg 2021;56(8):1405–10.
44. Howe AS, Vasudevan V, Kongnyuy M, et al. Degree of twisting and duration of symptoms are prognostic factors of testis salvage during episodes of testicular torsion. Transl Androl Urol 2017;6(6):1159–66.
45. Beni-Israel T, Goldman M, Bar Chaim S, et al. Clinical predictors for testicular torsion as seen in the pediatric ED. Am J Emerg Med 2010;28(7):786–9.
46. Liang T, Metcalfe P, Sevcik W, et al. Retrospective review of diagnosis and treatment in children presenting to the pediatric department with acute scrotum. AJR Am J Roentgenol 2013;200(5):W444–9.
47. Gaither T, Copp H. State appellant cases for testicular torsion: Case review from 1985 to 2015, J Pediatr Urol. 12 (5), 2016, e1-291
48. Chen M, Esler R. Accuracy and delay of using ultrasound in testicular torsion. J Urol Surg 2019;6:273–7.
49. Baker LA, Sigman D, Mathews RI, et al. An analysis of clinical outcomes using color doppler testicular ultrasound for testicular torsion. Pediatrics 2000;105: 604–7.
50. Boettcher M, Krebs T, Bergholz R, et al. Clinical and sonographic features predict testicular torsion in children: a prospective study. BJU Int 2013;112:1201–6.
51. Kravchick S, Cytron S, Leibovici O, et al. Color Doppler sonography: its real role in the evaluation of children with highly suspected testicular torsion. Eur Radiol 2001;11:1000–5.
52. Lam WW, Yap TL, Jacobsen AS, et al. Colour Doppler ultrasonography replacing surgical exploration for acute scrotum: myth or reality? Pediatr Radiol 2005;35: 597–600.
53. Xu Z, Wu J, Ni S, et al. The diagnostic value of ultrasound in pediatric testicular torsion with preserved flow. Front Pediatr 2022;10:1001958.
54. Blaivas M, Batts M, Lambert M. Ultrasonographic diagnosis of testicular torsion by emergency physicians. Am J Emerg Med 2000;18(2):198–200.
55. Russo T, Cozzi DA, Gaglione G, et al. The role of manual detorsion in pediatric testicular torsion during the global covid-19 pandemic: experience from 2 centres. Urology 2023;180:227–34.
56. Xu M, Hu L, Huang H, et al. Etiology and clinical features of full-term neonatal bacterial meningitis: a multicenter retrospective cohort study. Front Pediatr 2019;7:1–8.
57. Colaco M, Heavner M, Sunaryo P, et al. Malpractice litigation and testicular torsion: a legal database review. J Emerg Med 2015;49(6):849–54.
58. Aquila I, Abenavoli L, Sacco MA, et al. The limits of diagnosis of testicular torsion in the child: Medicolegal implications in clinical practice. Clin Case Rep 2021; 9(12):e05180.
59. Sawyer M., Enterovirus infections: Diagnosis and treatment. Semin Pediatr Infect Dis, 13, 2002, 40-7
60. Nigrovic LE, Kuppermann N, Malley R. Bacterial Meningitis Study Group of the Pediatric Emergency Medicine Collaborative Research Committee of the American Academy of Pediatrics, Children with bacterial meningitis presenting to the emergency department during the pneumococcal conjugate vaccine era. Acad Emerg Med 2008;15(6):522–8.
61. Hviid A, Melbye M. The epidemiology of viral meningitis hospitalization in childhood. Epidemiology 2007;18(6):695–701.

Chest Pain-Specific Legal Risk

Matthew DeLaney, MD*, Patrick Siler, MD

KEYWORDS

- Chest pain • Emergency medicine • Acute coronary syndrome
- Pulmonary embolism • Thoracic aortic dissection • Risk management

KEY POINTS

- Acute coronary syndromes, pulmonary emoblisms and aortic dissections account for the majority of chest pain related malpractice allegations.

Chest pain is one of the more common chief complaints in the emergency department (ED) accounting for over 10 million ED visits yearly resulting in an estimated cost of US$10 billion per year.[1] The emergency physician's differential diagnosis ranges from benign to acutely life-threatening etiologies with little distinction in how each might present. In addition to being an incredibly common chief complaint, chest pain-associated complaints are at the top for most common allegations of malpractice.[2]

In a retrospective analysis of over 6000 closed malpractice claims, Wong and colleagues found that when allegations of malpractice were made.[2] Approximately 66% of cases were dropped, dismissed, or withdrawn. Approximately 23% of the claims were settled with an average pay out of approximately US$300,000. For the 7.6% of cases that went to trial, the jury is generally sympathetic for the defense returning a verdict for the defendant in approximately 93% of cases. When the jury sided with the plaintiff, the average payout was approximately US$800,000.

Overall, cardiopulmonary conditions accounted for the majority of malpractice allegations with cardiac arrest (9.1%), acute myocardial infarction (4%), aortic aneurysm (2.3%), and pulmonary embolism (PE; 2.2%) being the most common conditions involved. In addition to being the most common sources of malpractice allegations, these cardiopulmonary conditions also had higher rates of claims being paid. When an allegation was made regarding malpractice associated with a myocardial infarction the paid–to–closed ratio was approximately 39%, which is well above the baseline rate reported for other conditions. The amount of money that was paid was notably

Department of Emergency Medicine, University of Alabama at Birmingham, 619 19th Street South, Birmingham, AL 35233, USA
* Corresponding author.
E-mail address: matthewcdelaney@gmail.com

Emerg Med Clin N Am 43 (2025) 57–65
https://doi.org/10.1016/j.emc.2024.05.025
0733-8627/25/© 2024 Elsevier Inc. All rights are reserved, including those for text and data mining, AI training, and similar technologies.
emed.theclinics.com

higher for allegations involving aortic aneurysms with an average payment of approximately US$370,000.[2]

In all closed claims, error in diagnosis was the most common chief medical error cited. Because of the commonality of chest pain as an ED complaint and the high medicolegal risk it poses, emergency medicine research is full of studies aiming to enhance the diagnostic precision, efficiency, and cost-effectiveness for the evaluation of chest pain.

Here, we will focus on the 3 most common missed diagnoses involved in malpractice allegations of patients with chest pain: acute coronary syndrome, PE, and thoracic aortic dissection (AD).

ACUTE CORONARY SYNDROME

Acute coronary syndrome (ACS) is a leading cause of death in the United States and also a source of significant medicolegal risk in the ED. Historically, the rate of missed myocardial infarctions has been thought to be as high as 8%; however, over the past few decades, the incidence of missed ACS is thought to be closer to 2% of patients discharged from the ED. While the overall rates of missed ACS seem to be decreasing, this subset of patients still carry a significant risk of adverse event following discharge with Pope and colleagues noting that discharged patients had almost twice the mortality of similar patients who were admitted for further observation and monitoring. In Pope's study, those discharged from the ED with ACS were more likely to be women aged under 55 years, non-White, those who reported shortness of breath as their chief complaint or had normal or nondiagnostic electrocardiograms.[3]

The presence of chest pain as a symptom is sensitive for ACS, but not particularly specific. In fact, there are few symptom differences between patients with ACS and those without ACS who present to the ED.[4] Several historical features have demonstrated some utility and thus should raise suspicion: pain that is described as similar to or worse than a previous myocardial infarction (MI), radiation to one or both arms, pain on exertion, vomiting and diaphoresis have all been shown to be predictive for ACS in some models.[5] It is also well documented that the accepted traditional risk factors for coronary artery disease do not predict an individual's risk to present with acute cardiac ischemia. According to Dezman and colleagues, history and physical alone are unable to reduce a patient's risk of ACS to the generally accepted level of 1% to 2%, arguing the evidence clearly shows that "atypical" symptoms cannot rule out ACS, while "typical" symptoms cannot rule ACS in. They ultimately conclude patients presenting with symptoms compatible with ACS likely warrant further ED investigation with electrocardiogram (ECG) and troponin measurement unless an alternative cause can be readily identified.[4]

The Electrocardiogram

With any suspicion higher than low probability for ACS, the ECG should not be the sole diagnostic tool used for evaluation. Physicians should have a low threshold to obtain serial ECGs in patients being evaluated for ACS; serial ECG utilization has been able to identify up to 16% of acute MIs not seen on initial presenting ECGs.[5] The miss rate of emergency physicians is similar to physicians of other specialties,[6] with a low incidence of clinically significant errors.[7,8]

The Troponin

For patients with more than a minimal risk, a troponin test will generally be done. Depending on the timing of the onset of pain (it needs to have been present long enough that the test will have turned positive) and if a conventional or high sensitivity troponin are being employed, 1 or 2 troponins can be done. Wassie and colleagues found that when a clinician used judgment in combination with the HEART score in deciding on 1 or 2 troponin tests, the second troponin was only positive 1 out of 200 times, there was no difference in outcomes; but most interestingly less than half of the clinicians ordered a second troponin… hard to say that ordering 2 troponins is standard of care (what a like or similarly trained clinician would do in a like or similar situation).[9]

In general, emergency physicians do a pretty good job of evaluating potential ACS. Review of claims data by the Insurance Committee of the American College of Emergency Physicians on missed MIs reveals that when we do miss, the patients were significantly younger, had less classic presentations, had fewer ECGs performed, and were seen by physicians with significantly less ED experience, who performed less thorough histories/documentation and were more prone to ECG misinterpretation.[10] Allegations of malpractice usually center around error in diagnosis or "failure to consider." More recently, risk stratification, diagnosis, and disposition in this patient population has been aided by the development of high-sensitivity troponin assays as well as validated, evidence-based decision tools such as the HEART pathway that when appropriately applied are able to identify a cohort at very low risk for adverse outcome.

PULMONARY EMBOLISM

PE is commonly seen in the ED and still accounts for a notable portion of chest pain-related allegations of malpractice. In an analysis of 277 malpractice cases involving PEs or deep vein thrombosis, Wilson and colleagues found that emergency physicians were involved in approximately 18% of the cases.[11] Overall, the most common suspected cause of PE was recent surgery, which accounted for 41% of the claims. In terms of the specific allegations of malpractice "failure to diagnose and treat" accounted for 62% of cases; 80% of cases involved an allegation of negligence that led to the patient's death. From a risk management standpoint, when these cases went to trial, the outcomes were different than what has been reported in other similar studies with only 16% of cases being settled prior to trial. When a verdict was returned, the jury sided with the defendant in only 57% of cases with 27% of cases ending in a verdict for the plaintiff. When a verdict was returned for the plaintiff, the median payout was approximately US$1,000,000 with a mean payout of approximately US$2,000,000.

One of the challenges associated with diagnosing PE is that patients often present atypically. In an analysis of data from the PIOPED II study, Stein and colleagues shed light on the variable presentations that can come from an underlying PE.[12] Unfortunately, a lot of the classic symptoms that we associate with PE were not seen in the majority of patients; only 44% of patients reported hemoptysis or pleuritic chest pain. New dyspnea either at rest or with exertion was the most common symptom and occurred in 73% of patients. Interestingly, most patients reported dyspnea at rest with only approximately 16% of patients having dyspnea only with exertion. Patients commonly reported that their dyspnea had a rapid onset, described as within seconds or minutes in over 80% of cases.

In terms of risk factors, 94% of patients had at least 1 risk factor for developing a PE with immobilization following surgery being the most common. Clinically, about 50% of the patients had tachypnea while only approximately 25% of patients were found to have tachycardia. While there is a clear association between the presence of a deep vein thrombosis and the presence of PE, only 32% of patients had any signs of calf swelling or pain. Though many patients did not have classic findings taught about PE, almost all (~98%) had dyspnea, tachypnea, pleuritic pain, or signs of deep vein thrombosis.

Making the diagnosis of PE when patients do not have classic symptoms remains a challenge. A case from 2015 sheds light on the current landscape associated with allegations of malpractice; in this high-profile case, a 15 year old patient was 1 week status postarthroscopic knee surgery and presented to the ED with a complaint of left chest pain that was noted to be worse when lying down. He denied fever and dyspnea, and he had normal vital signs. A chest radiograph and EKG were reported to be normal. He was diagnosed with pleurisy, administered a dose of ketorolac, and was sent home with a prescription for anti-inflammatories. Two weeks later the patient re-presented to the ED complaining of chest pain and dyspnea and unfortunately died from bilateral pulmonary emboli.

A malpractice case was filed, and the case ultimately went to trial. The plaintiffs hired a well-known high-profile emergency physician who claimed that on review of the chart that the patient had a "Q3T3" pattern on his EKG and signs of cardiomegaly on his radiograph—both of which allegedly were suggestive of an underlying PE. The plaintiff's experts claimed the care was "grossly improper, egregious, and contrary to well-known and fundamental medical principles." The jury returned a verdict for the plaintiff and agreed with the allegation that the physician was guilty of "gross negligence," which in Georgia has been defined as failing to provide a "slight" degree of medical care.[13] Interestingly, one of the plaintiff's experts was subsequently censured by the American College of Emergency Physicians regarding his testimony in this case.[14] This is consistent with the previously mentioned study by Wilson and colleagues, which found that 41% of the PE/deep vein thrombosis (DVT) malpractice cases had previous surgery.[12]

As with ACS from a risk management standpoint, the biggest allegations of malpractice related to PEs tends to be "failure to consider." Given the prevalence of PE and its associated rates of litigation when it is missed, it would be reasonable to consider it in any patients who have undifferentiated cardiopulmonary symptoms. While this may seem like a wide net to cast, when we use a structured approach to working up a potential PE, we are more accurate than when we rely on our bedside gestalt. In a retrospective analysis of over 1500 ED patients, Medson and colleagues found that "clinical hunch" or gestalt was associated with lower rates of PE diagnosis when compared to the pulmonary embolism rule out criteria (PERC) Rule, Wells score, revised Geneva score, and Years criteria.[15]

When it comes to making the decision to work up a patient, a common concern is that if we apply clinical decision tools and tests like a d-dimer, then we will end up unnecessarily testing a larger number of patients. While Hoo and colleagues found that the rate of computed tomography (CT) angiograms that were positive for PE increased from approximately 3% to approximately 16% after the Well's score and d-dimer was incorporated into the electronic health record, suggesting that this structured approach led to more appropriate use of testing and imaging.[16] There is an ongoing debate about the nuances of how to work up a potential PE, but as we see in this case, the big risk to both the patient and the clinician comes most often from failure to even *consider* the diagnosis rather than a missed diagnosis as a result of using a particular risk stratification system or particular brand of d-dimer. Even in a situation where PE is so unlikely that it would seem unnecessary to pursue any formal risk stratification simply documenting "PE would be highly unlikely because…" may offer a layer of medicolegal protection against allegations of "failure to consider."

AORTIC DISSECTION

While we have reliable and accurate ways to risk stratify patients who have potential ACS or PE to date, risk stratifying cases of potential AD remains challenging. From a medical standpoint, cases of AD are relatively rare, occurring in as few as 3 per 100,000 persons.[17] Another study showed that AD occurs in 1 out of 12,000 ED visits, 1 out of 980 chest pain visits to the point that the average full-time emergency physician would only see one case every 3 to 4 years.[18]

In addition to being seen only occasionally, cases of AD often present atypically as classic findings related to the historical elements and physical examination findings are not reliable and when studied have negative likelihood ratios that make it nearly impossible to rule out the diagnosis based on the history or physical examination. Even classic radiographic findings such as a widened mediastinum on chest radiograph does little to move the diagnostic needle. More recently, risk stratification tools such as the AD detection risk score have been developed—but not surprisingly, these too struggle to offer reliable diagnostic clarity.[19] Cases of AD can present a medico-legal perfect storm as they present sporadically, atypically, and are difficult to diagnose at the bedside. It has been said that "...when dealing with AD the standard of care may be to miss it on the first visit," a statement that while likely accurate does not offer any practical advice in terms of risk management.[20]

In a retrospective analysis of 109 ED patients who were diagnosed with acute AD, Kurabayashi and colleagues found that approximately 60% of patients were misdiagnosed during their initial assessment in the ED.[21] When the patient was misdiagnosed, it was thought that they were having ACS in approximately 63% of cases. Clinically, patients who are misdiagnosed have some unique characteristics. When patients arrived via ambulance, the misdiagnoses rate was 10% compared to 29% in patients who presented via private vehicle. Anterior chest pain is present in 71% of cases that were initially misdiagnosed versus 41% of cases who are correctly identified as having an underlying AD. On radiograph, a widened mediastinum was seen in only 25% of cases where the patient was misdiagnosed versus 55% of cases when a correct diagnosis was made. Overall patients who were misdiagnosed had approximately half the imaging studies as patients who were correctly diagnosed. Interestingly, despite this rate of missed diagnosis, there is no statistical difference in regard to in-hospital mortality (18% vs 15%, $P = .520$).

Palaniappan and colleagues reviewed 135 malpractice cases involving AD. Overall, 23% of cases were settled. When the case went to trial, the jury returned with a defense verdict in 57% of cases while siding with the plaintiff 20% of the time.[22] There were significant differences in terms of the specific allegations of malpractice when a jury sided for the defense versus the plaintiff. In cases where a defense verdict was returned, the most common allegations were failure to test, failure to refer, and failure to consult in the presence of a stroke. When the plaintiff verdict was returned, the most common allegation was failure to diagnose. In terms of payouts, in cases where a patient died, the amount paid on average was less than the amount paid when a patient survived (~US$1,800,000 vs ~US$5,900,000). This may seem counterintuitive but likely is an accurate reflection of the patient population involved in these cases. On average, patients with missed AD are going to be elderly and have an associated lower monetary value given their life expectancy and reduced potential for lost wages. Alternatively, a patient who survives a missed AD likely has ongoing costs associated with their alleged damages and may have a higher overall economic burden.

While specific features of the patient's clinical presentation in isolation do not necessarily help us identify patients who have an underlying AD, a retrospective analysis of cases of AD by Ohle and colleagues suggests that having a structured approach to patients with a potential AD may help decrease the rates of misdiagnosis.[23] In a review of 194 cases of AD, Ohle and colleagues found that the rate of misdiagnosis was 17.6%. Cases were reviewed to see how many "pain descriptors" were asked and documented. These questions included severity, abrupt onset of pain, radiating pain, general character of pain, and duration of pain. When comparing cases of missed diagnosis versus those of correct diagnosis, severity of pain and duration of pain are asked more often in cases where the correct diagnosis was made. Overall, the study argued that simply gathering additional data by asking more questions can be associated with a lower risk of missed diagnosis. When less than 2 questions were asked, the rate of misdiagnosis was about 20%, which was approximately 4 times higher than was noted in cases where greater than 2 questions were asked. While the study does not give us a clear pathway to reliably reduce the rate of missed diagnosis, it does suggest that simply stopping and thinking about the potential of AD and obtaining a more thorough history may, in fact, reduce the risk of missed diagnosis.

From a risk management standpoint, it is difficult to eliminate the medicolegal risk associated with cases of missed AD. Unlike in the case of ACS and PE where we have validated widely accepted risk stratification tools, short of ordering CT angiography on every patient with chest pain, it is difficult to accurately determine if the patient with nondescript chest pain in the ED has an AD. A recent clinical policy of the American College of Emergency Physicians shed light on the challenging nature of this disease process, finding largely low-quality evidence without identifying a reliable way to rule out the presence of an underlying AD short of getting definitive imaging with angiography.[24] Charting the absence or presence of classic features can buffer against allegations of failure to consider. Unfortunately, cases of missed AD will likely continue to be a rare but significant source of risk to both the patient and the clinician.

RISK MANAGEMENT AT THE BEDSIDE

While no amount of charting can completely prevent a lawsuit given the prevalence of malpractice cases associated with complaints of chest pain, it is reasonable to develop a consistent and concise approach to documenting these encounters. As discussed earlier, the main allegation for ACS, PE, and AD is "failure to consider" the diagnosis. For any cases of undifferentiated chest pain, simply stating "Based on the clinical picture, low risk of ACS, PE, and AD" undoubtedly offers a first line of defense against allegations of malpractice. Beyond this simple broad approach, risk stratification using and documenting an established risk stratification tool such as the HEART score provides an additional layer of protection. A final layer of documentation protection can occur when a clinician identifies potential red flags. For example, if a triage note documents that a patient has tearing/ripping chest pain that radiates to their back it would be reasonable to document why this is *not* concerning for AD and also explicitly stating that you do not think the patient needs definitive testing for evaluation. While there are no clear best practices as to the specifics of documentation, a strong chart would convey the sense that the clinician took the patient seriously, considered the big 3 (ACS, AD, and PE), and made the best decision they could using the available evidence. At the end of the day, failure to make the diagnosis does not necessarily mean that a case has deviated from the standard of care as often when cases are litigated, being able to show a jury that the treating team tried their best to help the patient is generally very supportive to the defense.

Over the past decade, there has been an increased use of shared medical decision-making (SDM) when helping to determine next steps in the treatment and disposition of patients in the ED with chest pain. On the surface, SDM would seem to lessen the clinician's degree of medicolegal risk as the patient is helping to determine their next steps, yet there is concern that when used incorrectly SDM may actually *increase* a clinician's potential risk. In theory, SDM must offer the patient a choice between reasonable alternative pathways and be made with clinician guidance.

An ideal situation would be a scenario where a patient with a HEART score of 4 chooses to go home with close follow-up rather than be admitted, as both options seem reasonable based on the current medical literature. Alternatively, in a case a patient with a HEART score of 7 was discharged home and ultimately had a bad outcome. When the case was reviewed, the note stated, "SDM was conducted and the patient chose to go home." This case seems to stretch the concept of SDM to a degree that it actually draws the quality of the care into question. Given current literature, discharging a patient home with a HEART score of 7 would not likely be considered to be a reasonable next step. Obviously, there are situations where a patient could choose to go home with a HEART score of 7, but arguably this would involve the patient making a choice to act against what would be standard medical advice. In these situations, patients should be categorized and documented as leaving against medical advice (AMA) rather than leaving after SDM. While this may seem like mere semantics, the distinctions between these 2 designations can be rather significant.

When a patient leaves AMA, the courts have consistently recognized a patient's right to make decisions that would go against standard medical advice. While an AMA discharge does not eliminate the medicolegal risk, it does lower it significantly—in particular, if the clinician can document the discussion and decision making as well as establish that the patient was aware of the risks, had capacity, and still decided to leave. In the case of a patient with a heart score of 7, rather than reducing the clinician's risk, the term SDM could be used to argue that the clinician in fact gave the patient the option of making a high-risk choice.

SUMMARY

It is difficult to work a shift in the ED without seeing a patient with chest pain. Unfortunately, mixed in with the masses of benign chest pain patients, there are time bombs of ACS, PE, and AD that may evolve into malpractice cases. While consistently considering and appropriately risk stratifying for these big 3 ominous causes of chest pain may improve patient outcomes and reduce the medicolegal risk—these steps alone do not eliminate the rare case that slips through. The best approach to minimizing risk is to gather appropriate data and to explain your thought process as to why you do *not* think one of the "big 3" are occurring, but nothing is 100%. A seasoned defense lawyer once remarked, "The most important thing to remember at the end of the day is that you need to keep paying the premiums on your malpractice insurance."

CLINICS CARE POINTS

- It is crucial to consider the risk of ACS, PE, and AD in any patient who presents to the emergency department with chest pain.

DISCLOSURE

The authors have no financial disclosures or conflicts of interest.

REFERENCES

1. American College of Emergency Physicians Clinical Policies Subcommittee (Writing Committee) on Suspected Non–ST-Elevation Acute Coronary Syndromes:, Tomaszewski CA, Nestler D, Shah KH, et al. Clinical Policy: Critical Issues in the Evaluation and Management of Emergency Department Patients With Suspected Non-ST-Elevation Acute Coronary Syndromes. Ann Emerg Med 2018;72(5):e65–106. PMID: 30342745.

2. Wong KE, Parikh PD, Miller KC, et al. Emergency Department and Urgent Care Medical Malpractice Claims 2001-15. West J Emerg Med 2021;22(2):333–8. PMID: 33856320; PMCID: PMC7972370.

3. Pope JH, Selker HP. Acute coronary syndromes in the emergency department: diagnostic characteristics, tests, and challenges. Cardiol Clin 2005;23(4): 423–51, v-vi.

4. Dezman ZD, Mattu A, Body R. Utility of the history and physical examination in the detection of acute coronary syndromes in emergency department patients. West J Emerg Med 2017;18(4):752–60. Epub 2017 May 3. PMID: 28611898; PMCID: PMC5468083.

5. Fesmire FM, Percy RF, Bardoner JB, et al. Usefulness of automated serial 12-lead ECG monitoring during the initial emergency department evaluation of patients with chest pain. Ann Emerg Med 1998;31:3–11.

6. McCabe JM, Armstrong EJ, Ku I, et al. Physician accuracy in interpreting potential ST-segment elevation myocardial infarction electrocardiograms. J Am Heart Assoc 2013;2(5):e000268.

7. Snoey ER, Housset B, Guyon P, et al. Analysis of emergency department interpretation of electrocardiograms. J Accid Emerg Med 1994;11(3):149–53.

8. Todd KH, Hoffman JR, Morgan MT. Effect of cardiologist ECG review on emergency department practice. Ann Emerg Med 1996;27(1):16–21.

9. Wassie M, Lee MS, Sun BC, et al. Single vs serial measurements of cardiac troponin level in the evaluation of patients in the emergency department with suspected acute myocardial infarction. JAMA Netw Open 2021;4(2):e2037930.

10. Rusnak RA, Stair TO, Hansen K, et al. Litigation against the emergency physician: common features in cases of missed myocardial infarction. Ann Emerg Med 1989;18:102934.

11. Wilson E, Phair J, Carnevale M, et al. Common reasons for malpractice lawsuits involving pulmonary embolism and deep vein thrombosis. J Surg Res 2020;245: 212–6. Epub 2019 Aug 14. PMID: 31421365.

12. Stein PD, Beemath A, Matta F, et al. Clinical characteristics of patients with acute pulmonary embolism: data from PIOPED II. Am J Med 2007;120(10):871–9. PMID: 17904458; PMCID: PMC2071924.

13. van Meerten K.F., Haan R.M.A., Dekker I.M.C., et al., The interobserver agreement of the HEART-score, a multicentre prospective study. Eur J Emerg Med. 2021;28(2):111-118. Available at: http://caselaw.findlaw.com/ga-court-of-appeals/1616486.html, Accessed April 27, 2024.

14. ACEP Issues, Available at: https://www.acepnow.com/article/acep-issues-public-censure/. Accessed April 27, 2024.

15. Medson K, Yu J, Liwenborg L, et al. Comparing 'clinical hunch' against clinical decision support systems (PERC rule, wells score, revised Geneva score and YEARS criteria) in the diagnosis of acute pulmonary embolism. BMC Pulm Med 2022;22(1):432. PMID: 36414971; PMCID: PMC9682736.

16. Hoo GW, Wu CC, Vazirani S, et al. Does a clinical decision rule using D-dimer level improve the yield of pulmonary CT angiography? AJR Am J Roentgenol 2011;196(5):1059–64. PMID: 21512071.
17. Clouse WD, Hallett JW Jr, Schaff HV, et al. Acute aortic dissection: population-based incidence compared with degenerative aortic aneurysm rupture. Mayo Clin Proc 2004;79(2):176–80. PMID: 14959911.
18. Alter SM, Eskin B, Allegra JR. Diagnosis of aortic dissection in emergency department patients is rare. West J Emerg Med 2015;16(5):629–31.
19. Nazerian P, Pivetta E, Veglia S, et al. Integrated use of conventional chest radiography cannot rule out acute aortic syndromes in emergency department patients at low clinical probability. Acad Emerg Med 2019;26(11):1255–65. Epub 2019 Jul 22. PMID: 31220387.
20. Elefteriades JA, Barrett PW, Kopf GS. Litigation in nontraumatic aortic diseases–a tempest in the malpractice maelstrom. Cardiology 2008;109(4):263–72.
21. Kurabayashi M, Miwa N, Ueshima D, et al. Factors leading to failure to diagnose acute aortic dissection in the emergency room. J Cardiol 2011;58(3):287–93. Epub 2011 Sep 3. PMID: 21889877.
22. Palaniappan A, Sellke F. Medical malpractice litigations involving aortic dissection. J Thorac Cardiovasc Surg 2022;164(2):600–8. Epub 2020 Oct 29. PMID: 33229180.
23. Ohle R, Mc IS, Perry JJ. A simple intervention to reduce your chance of missing an acute aortic dissection. CJEM 2019;21(5):618–21. PMID: 30907334.
24. American College of Emergency Physicians Clinical Policies Subcommittee (Writing Committee) on Thoracic Aortic Dissection, Diercks DB, Promes SB, Schuur JD, et al. Clinical policy: critical issues in the evaluation and management of adult patients with suspected acute nontraumatic thoracic aortic dissection. Ann Emerg Med 2015;65(1):32–42.e12. Erratum in: Ann Emerg Med. 2017 Nov;70(5):758. PMID: 25529153.

Misdiagnosis of Acute Headache
Mitigating Medico-legal Risks

Jonathan A. Edlow, MD[a,b,*]

KEYWORDS

- Acute headache • Thunderclap headache • Misdiagnosis
- Subarachnoid hemorrhage • Physical examination

KEY POINTS

- Use details of the history to identify red flags that suggest serious causes of headache.
- Remember that in thunderclap headache, there are other serious causes beyond subarachnoid hemorrhage.
- Apply a targeted physical examination to further refine possible red flags.
- Understand the limitations of imaging tests.
- Always document your medical-decision-making to show your thought process.

INTRODUCTION AND METHODS

Headache is a common presenting complaint in the emergency department (ED).[1] In the general population, primary headache disorders—migraine and tension-type headache—are incredibly common. Approximately 12% of the population has migraine headaches.[2] The 1 year US prevalence is 47 million individuals with migraine and 65.6 million with tension-type headache.[3] Most do not seek care in the ED, but migraine is still a common reason for ED visits. By contrast, secondary headache disorders are orders-of-magnitude less common, setting up the familiar emergency medicine conundrum of the needle in the haystack.

Whereas knowledge about migraine is important for emergency clinicians,[4] a missed migraine diagnosis does not have the same medico-legal implications than missing a subarachnoid hemorrhage (SAH) or a vertebral artery dissection. This article reviews diagnosis and misdiagnosis of secondary headaches in the ED. The author also proposes some practical methods to avoid or mitigate the effects of misdiagnosis based on a non-systematic literature search, my 40 years of clinical experience, my 25 years of attendance of weekly morbidity and mortality conferences, and over 20 years of experience reviewing medical malpractice cases for both defense and plaintiff firms.

[a] Department of Emergency Medicine, Harvard Medical School, Boston, MA, USA; [b] Emergency Medicine, Beth Israel Deaconess Medical Center, Boston, MA, USA
* 313 Paynes Creek Road, Lancaster, VA 22503
E-mail address: jedlow@bidmc.harvard.edu

Emerg Med Clin N Am 43 (2025) 67–80
https://doi.org/10.1016/j.emc.2024.05.026
0733-8627/25/© 2024 Elsevier Inc. All rights are reserved, including those for text and data mining, AI training, and similar technologies.
emed.theclinics.com

"CANNOT MISS" CAUSES OF ACUTE HEADACHE

Not every patient with a headache requires a specific etiologic diagnosis. The distinction between migraine and tension-type headache[4] is not necessary given the usual "rules of engagement" in emergency medicine—to diagnose and treat serious conditions that threaten life, limb, brain, or vision. **Box 1** lists "cannot miss" diagnoses (conditions that are diagnosable in the ED and have time-sensitive treatments without which, bad outcomes are more likely).

It is neither necessary nor wise to perform tests to rule out all of these conditions in every patient with headache. Increased availability and use of imaging for many conditions does not necessarily improve diagnostic accuracy, either because the test is used in the wrong patients,[5] or its limitations are not understood.[6] Nonetheless, there is benefit to mentally running through this differential diagnostic checklist in patients with headache because many of these conditions can be easily discarded based on clinical evaluation alone. For example, giant cell arteritis (GCA) is not a serious consideration in a 40 year old individual. SAH would be highly unlikely in a patient whose headache has gradually worsened over 3 days. Acute narrow angle closure glaucoma (ANAG) would be extraordinarily unlikely in a patient with a normal eye examination.

MISDIAGNOSIS, MISCONCEPTIONS, AND RED FLAGS

That said, there is considerable overlap in headache characteristics between primary headaches and secondary ones; therefore, "cannot miss" diagnoses cannot be excluded by clinical evaluation alone. For example, the majority of patients

---

Box 1
Differential diagnosis of "cannot miss" causes of acute headache

Vascular conditions
    Subarachnoid hemorrhage
    Reversible cerebral vasoconstriction syndrome
    Ischemic stroke
    Hemorrhagic stroke
    Cervical artery dissection
    Cerebral venous sinus thrombosis
    Hypertensive crisis
    Posterior reversible encephalopathy syndrome
    Giant cell arteritis

Infections causes
    Meningitis
    Encephalitis
    Brain abscess
    Epidural empyema

Mass lesions
    Tumors and cysts
    Subdural and epidural hematoma
    Pituitary apoplexy
    Abscess and empyema

CSF pressure-related causes
    Idiopathic intracranial hypertension
    Spontaneous intracranial hypotension

Miscellaneous
    Carbon monoxide poisoning
    Narrow angle closure glaucoma

with thunderclap headaches have primary headache syndromes,[7] and only a small minority of patients with cerebral venous sinus thrombosis (CVST),[8,9] or cervical artery dissection,[10] have thunderclap headaches. Only a minority of patients with brain tumor have the "classic" headaches that are worse in the morning or with cough.[11]

"Textbook" or "classic" descriptions are rarely the most common. Of 668 patients with brain abscess, only 20% had that classic triad (fever, headache, and focal neurological deficits).[12] The classic teaching that patients with acute onset deficits in both balance and hearing indicates that a peripheral process is incorrect; strokes of the anterior inferior cerebellar artery or its branches also present this way.[13]

Red flags—specific patient or symptom characteristics that drive a diagnostic evaluation beyond history and physical examination—are helpful in the diagnosis of acute headache.[14–17] **Table 1** lists these red flags. Using red flags is nothing more than applying basic principles of history-taking, physical examination, and the process of differential diagnosis to decide on what further diagnostic testing (if any) is justified for an individual patient. These red flags prioritize sensitivity over specificity. Because the sensitivity for most single red flags is low, combinations of them probably perform better.

REASONS FOR MISDIAGNOSIS AND STRATEGIES TO AVOID OR MITIGATE THEM BY PROCESS OF CARE
History

Patients and clinicians often use terms such as "migraine" or "sinus" headache indiscriminately. Some patients describe any severe headache as a "migraine," a word that is sometimes incorporated into the triage note as "past medical history," which can lead to diagnostic anchoring. There is a distinction between patients labeling their headache a "migraine" and a diagnosis of migraine made by a neurologist. Another common example is that frontal pain over the sinuses is often referred to as a "sinus headache," but sinus headaches are actually uncommon.[18] Both situations can lead to incorrect diagnoses.

Key elements of the history of a patient with a headache include the mode of onset (sudden, "thunderclap" vs gradual), pain duration, and evolution overtime. In reviewing malpractice cases, it is surprising how often the simple element of onset is missing, even though it is so easy to obtain and is actionable. All thunderclap headaches need a work-up. Some have questioned the definition of thunderclap headache as one that starts and reaches maximal intensity within 1 minute.[19] In one prospective study that included 132 patients with SAH, 6 (4.5%) had time from onset to peak intensity was 1 hour.[20] For this reason, I not rigidly apply the 1 minute definition.

Although SAH is the most notorious cause of thunderclap headache, reversible cerebral vasoconstriction syndrome (RCVS) is just as common a cause in ED populations, each comprising approximately 8% of cases of thunderclap headache.[21–23] **Table 2** lists the causes of thunderclap headache.[7,24]

By definition, migraine headaches last less than 72 hours.[25] Progressive increased intensity overtime is worrisome. However, longer the duration of a headache, the less likely it is due to a serious cause.[17,26] In one study of 118 patients with brain tumors, the longest duration of headache was 77 days, suggesting that headache that has lasted more than several months is unlikely to be due to a tumor.[27] There are 2 exceptions to this general principle about duration. ANAG often presents with episodes of headache lasting minutes to a few hours that go undiagnosed for years before correct diagnosis.[28] Visual symptoms may be absent. Colloid cyst of the third ventricle is another very rare condition that can present with intermittent episodes of severe headache over years.[29,30] Episodes are often associated with vomiting and relieved by lying down.

Table 1
Red flags and situations suggesting the need for evaluation beyond history and physical examination

Red Flag	Significance
History—headache characteristics	
Onset	Rapid (thunderclap) onset suggests a specific group of diagnoses, most notably SAH and RCVS
Evolution overtime	Progressive increase over days or weeks
Headache worsens with standing up	Spontaneous intracranial hypotension (or post-dural puncture headache)
Headache worsens with lying down, cough, or Valsalva	Brain tumor, Chiari malformation
Other neurologic symptoms also present	Serious secondary diagnoses
Recent head or neck trauma	Subdural hematoma or arterial dissection
History of fever	Meningitis, encephalitis, brain abscess, or subdural empyema
Changes in preexisting headache pattern	Any secondary cause in a patient with a preexisting primary headache diagnosis
Epidemiologic context	
Increasing age	ICH, GCA
History of systemic cancer	Metastatic tumor
Pregnant or postpartum	RCVS, CVST, PRES, preeclampsia/eclampsia, post-dura puncture headache, pituitary apoplexy
Immunocompromised state	Opportunistic infections
Hypercoagulable state	Cerebral venous sinus thrombosis
Obesity and female sex	Idiopathic intracranial hypertension
Anticoagulant use	ICH
Clustering of multiple cases	Carbon monoxide poisoning
Recent lumbar puncture	Post-dural puncture headache
Known pituitary adenoma	Pituitary apoplexy
Family history of cerebral aneurysms or SAH	SAH
Physical examination	
Fever on examination	Same as history of fever
Hypertension	Hypertensive crisis, PRES, anything causing high ICP
Abnormal temporal artery	GCA
Meningismus	Meningitis or SAH
Any new neurologic deficit	Any secondary cause
Horner's syndrome	Carotid dissection, Wallenberg syndrome
Extraocular muscles	Third nerve palsy—aneurysm, sixth nerve palsy—elevated ICP or IIH
Pupils and eye examination	PCom, ANAG, Horner's
Fundoscopic examination (or abnormal ONSD on ultrasound)	Papilledema or absent venous pulsations—elevated ICH, subhyaloid hemorrhage—SAH or ICH

Abbreviations: ANAG, acute narrow-angle glaucoma; CVST, cerebral venous sinus thrombosis; GCA, giant cell arteritis; ICH, intracranial hemorrhage; ICP, intracranial pressure; ONSD, optic nerve sheath diameter; PCom, posterior communicating artery; PRES, posterior reversible encephalopathy syndrome; RCVS, reversible cerebral vasoconstriction syndrome; SAH, subarachnoid hemorrhage.

Note: Some authors have suggested SNOOP$_4$ to as an aid to remembering headache red flags.

S, systemic infection, secondary diseases; N, neurologic symptoms and signs; O, Onset; O, Older age (>50 years); P1, Positional; P2, Prior history; P3, Pregnancy/postpartum; P4, Precipitated by Valsalva.

Table 2
Causes of thunderclap headache

Condition	Comments
Common Causes	
Subarachnoid hemorrhages	Can be isolated headache or neck pain, often with vomiting or transient loss of consciousness. Overall, 40% will have headache with an otherwise normal physical examination
Reversible cerebral vasoconstriction syndrome[a]	Multiple short-duration (several hours) thunderclap headaches, usually with some precipitating trigger. Physical examination may be normal
Migraine, cluster headache, and primary thunderclap headache[a]	These are diagnoses of exclusion that should never be made without an extensive evaluation for secondary causes
Uncommon causes	
Arterial dissection[a]	Occurs in ~ 3% to 5% of carotid dissections and ~ 10% of vertebral dissections. Physical examination may be normal
Cerebral venous sinus thrombosis[a]	Occurs in ~ 10% of venous sinus thromboses. Physical examination may be normal
Acute stroke[a]	Can occur with ischemic (usually posterior circulation) or hemorrhagic stroke. Usually with a neurologic deficit
Acute subdural hematoma	Other findings are usually present
Retroclival hematoma	Cranial neuropathies may be present
Hypertensive encephalopathy[a]	Associated with elevated blood pressure and evidence of end-organ dysfunction (not any specific blood pressure)
Posterior reversible encephalopathy syndrome[a]	Usually not thunderclap. A seizure precedes the headache. Visual symptoms are common. Most cases have hypertension
Preeclampsia/eclampsia[a]	Can occur postpartum
Pituitary apoplexy[a]	Often in setting of a preexisting pituitary adenoma, often with ophthalmoplegia and bitemporal hemianopsia. Physical examination may be normal.
Spontaneous intracranial hypotension[a]	Thunderclap headache in ~ 15% of cases. Headache is usually positional (worse standing, better lying down).
Sphenoid sinusitis	
Rare causes, mostly described in isolated case reports	
Meningitis or encephalitis	
Unruptured aneurysm[a]	Rare, from acute expansion, thrombosis or dissection of a preexisting aneurysm
Colloid cyst of the third ventricle	Often a history of multiple prior headaches over years
Spontaneous retroclival hematoma	
Giant cell arteritis[a]	
Myocardial infarction[a]	
Aortic dissection[a]	

[a] These causes may be associated with a normal non-contrast brain CT scan and lumbar puncture depending on timing of CT (ischemic stroke) or if the opening pressure is measured on the lumbar puncture (spontaneous intracranial hypotension).

Pain intensity and location are, by themselves, less important diagnostic factors. Exacerbating and alleviating factors suggest specific diagnoses. Headaches that worsen with standing and are relieved by lying down suggest low-pressure headaches (post-dural puncture or spontaneous intracranial hypotension), whereas headaches that are exacerbated by cough, Valsalva, or the recumbent position suggest elevated intracranial pressure (ICP).[14] One uncommon cause of headaches precipitated by cough is a Chiari malformation.[31]

Every patient with headache "plus" (headache plus other new neurologic symptoms, such as seizure, visual abnormalities, weakness, and diplopia) needs sufficient work-up to identify the cause of those "plus" symptoms.

Elderly patients can develop a subdural hematoma after trivial head trauma, due to tearing of taut bridging veins that traverse the widened space between the inner table of the skull and the surface of an atrophic brain. Patients with dementia or alcohol-use disorder may fall and not remember and have a chronic subdural hematoma. Anticoagulated patients with minimal head trauma and even without loss of consciousness or visible evidence of injury may still have an intracranial hemorrhage (ICH).[32] These patients usually have headaches, often accompanied by weakness, personality change, or other new symptoms. Recent minor head or neck trauma can also cause arterial dissections. Patients with headache and fever may have any of a number of infectious conditions, some involving the central nervous system.

Finally, it is important to be aware that because primary headache disorders are so common, migraineurs can develop secondary causes that manifest as a change in the typical pattern of their headaches. Questions that may be helpful to differentiate exacerbation of a chronic migraine versus a more serious cause include

"How often do you get your migraines?"

"How often do you come to the ED for them?"

"Does this current headache differ from your usual migraine?"

"Do you have any additional symptoms now that you usually do not have?"

One should be exceptionally cautious about diagnosing "complex migraine" in the ED unless the patient has had multiple prior similar episodes over a long period of time that have been properly evaluated.

Epidemiologic Context

Because development of a new primary headache disorder decreases with age and because some of the serious secondary causes become more common, increasing age is identified as a red flag for secondary causes. Studies have defined "elderly" differently, the lowest one being 50 years. The 2008 American College of Emergency Physicians (ACEP) clinical policy on headache has a low-grade recommendation to "consider" urgent brain imaging in patients older than 50 years,[33] but there is obviously no hard and fast cut point. Specific pathologies to consider are subdural hematoma following minor trauma, and GCA. As a general rule, in patients over the age of 50 years with a new headache and no clear explanation, I recommend sending off inflammatory biomarkers, preferably both C-reactive protein (CRP) and erythrocyte sedimentation rate if both are available.[34,35]

Patients with a history of a systemic cancer are at risk for brain metastases, even years after remission. Although migraine is still the most common cause of headache in pregnant or postpartum women, they are at higher risk for preeclampsia, eclampsia, CVST, posterior reversible encephalopathy syndrome (PRES), RCVS, post-dural puncture headache (after a spinal anesthetic), spontaneous intracranial hypotension (from labor-related pushing causing a dural tear), and pituitary apoplexy.[36–38] Many of these conditions require advanced imaging with either MRI (PRES or intracranial hypotension)[39] or computed tomographic angiography (CTA)/computed tomographic venography (CTV) (CVST and RCVS). ACEP guidelines recommend brain imaging in immunocompromised patients with headache.[33] Cryptococcal meningitis is another concern in this group. Patients who are fully anticoagulated are at higher risk for ICH.

Physical Examination

Fever suggests the possibility of meningitis, encephalitis, brain abscess, and epidural empyema although only half of patients with brain abscess have fever.[12] Hypertension suggests hypertensive emergency (hypertensive crisis), PRES, or it may be a compensatory mechanism to preserve cerebral blood flow in any condition associated with elevated ICP. Of course, it could also be related to pain or anxiety, but one should not assume this to be the cause.

The general examination might show temporal artery redness, tenderness, swelling, or nodularity consistent with GCA. Meningismus, the presence of palpable resistance when the neck is passively flexed, suggests meningeal irritation due to the presence of blood (SAH) or pus (meningitis).

A thorough neurologic examination should be done. Any new abnormality should be explained. Although their presence does not absolutely mean that there is a secondary cause,[40] it is a safe practice to assume that they do, unless the patient has had multiple similar episodes of headache with the finding over a months to years. On the other hand, serious secondary causes of headache can occur with a completely normal examination, and even when that examination is done by neurologists.[41]

The cranial nerves and eye examinations can be diagnostically useful. A third cranial nerve palsy, especially if associated with a dilated pupil, suggests an aneurysm of the posterior communicating artery. However, a sixth nerve palsy is often non-localizing and is seen with elevated ICP including idiopathy intracranial hypertension or low ICP (spontaneous intracranial hypotension). Cranial nerve findings can also be associated with indolent forms of meningitis that present with headache including meningitis due to Lyme disease,[42] cryptococcus,[43] tuberculosis,[44] carcinomatosis,[45] and others.[46]

An abnormally small pupil suggests a Horner's syndrome, which is found in half of patients with carotid dissections.[10] In ANAG, in addition to a fixed mid-position pupil, the eye is red with a limbal flush and a "steamy" edematous cornea. Intraocular pressure is elevated.

Performing fundoscopy in ED patients with headache is best practice. Papilledema and the absence of venous pulsations suggest elevated ICP and retinal subhyaloid hemorrhages are found in approximately 10% of cases of SAH. In my experience of routinely looking for venous pulsations then measuring the opening pressure directly on lumbar puncture (LP), I have only encountered 2 patients with normal venous pulsations but whose measured pressure was elevated (neither of which was markedly elevated).

Although fundoscopy used to be standard practice, skills and confidence in interpreting fundoscopy have declined.[47] In the international HEAD study of 4536 ED patients with nontraumatic headache, ophthalmoscopy was only performed in 7% of patients.[48] Some have begun to question its utility in the ED.[49] Practically speaking, while ophthalmoscopy may be best practice and is very useful in patients with idiopathic intracranial hypertension (IIH; pseudotumor cerebri) or other causes of raised ICP, it can no longer be considered "standard."

Another method of estimating ICP is measuring the optic nerve sheath diameter (ONSD) by ultrasound. A meta-analysis found that ONSD had both excellent sensitivity and specificity for ICP compared to computed tomographic (CT) scanning.[50] The ONSD changes in real time compared to opening and closing pressures measured by LP in patients with IIH (pseudotumor cerebri).[51,52] Increasing data show that non-mydriatic retinal photography can be diagnostically useful in the ED,[53,54] although this is not widely available.

Practically speaking, while ophthalmoscopy may be best practice, it is no longer standard.

Brain and Cerebrovascular Imaging

Brain imaging does not need to be performed on every ED patient with headache. In the HEAD study, CT was performed in 37% of patients with wide variation from country to country.[48] But which patients should have imaging and what type?

Non-contrast CT has excellent sensitivity for acute bleeding, and most symptomatic brain tumors and other mass lesions, but will miss many of the diagnoses on the "cannot miss" list. Concluding that there is no serious pathology after a negative CT scan is a common scenario in malpractice cases regarding headache. For example, in CVST, the sensitivity of non-contrast CT is less than 80%.[55,56] MRI is far more sensitive for most causes of headache (including ICH). No matter which study is ordered, communicate your diagnostic concerns to the radiologist rather than simply writing "headache" on the requisition. Of course, both CT and MRI will be negative for many serious causes without structural damage including carbon monoxide poisoning, GCA, ANAG, arterial dissection, eclampsia, meningitis/encephalitis, and IIH (pseudotumor cerebri).

Another trap is concluding that a "positive" CT showing an incidental radiographic finding is the etiology of the headache. The common finding of mucosal thickening documented in the radiologist's report as chronic "sinusitis" can be incorrectly interpreted by the clinician that sinusitis is the cause of the headache; however, the conclusion that the finding (musical thickening) is the cause of the headache is usually wrong.[57] This same lack of causality may be true for other incidental findings including small meningiomas or calcifications in the basal ganglia.

CT angiography is often done now in place of lumbar puncture for query SAH. This is very sensitive for aneurysms but does not diagnose SAH and has some negative downstream consequences inherent to overtesting.[58] CTA is also very sensitive for arterial dissections, RCVS (after the first week), and the vascular cause of various etiologies of ICH. The venous phase will usually show CVST for which CTV is diagnostically equivalent to magnetic resonance venography (MRV).[59]

Laboratory Testing

Routine laboratory testing of blood and urine is rarely useful in patients with acute headache, but important exceptions include inflammatory markers in question GCA, "eclampsia laboratories" for preeclampsia and co-oximetry for possible carbon monoxide poisoning.

Lumbar Puncture and Cerebrospinal Fluid Analysis

The LP is not dead. Cerebrospinal fluid (CSF) analysis remains a unique way of examining patients' ICP, cell counts, protein levels, and others. Ideally, the procedure should be done in the recumbent position so that an accurate opening pressure can be measured. The common practice of having the patient relax and extend their legs has not been shown to significantly reduce the pressures.[60] It may, however, help the patient be more comfortable. In patients with obesity, ultrasound-guided LP can reduce the time to complete the procedure and increase the success rate.[61]

Measuring opening pressure with a manometer is the most accurate way to know the ICP in the ED. The normal opening pressure ranges from 6 to 25 cm of water. If the LP has to be done sitting up, after obtaining the CSF, slowly reposition the patient to the side-lying position and measure the closing pressure. Differentiating a traumatic tap from true SAH can often be accomplished by wasting 5 to 10 cc between tubes 1 and 4 to reduce the red blood cell count in the last tube, often, to 0 (or close to 0) if the tap is traumatic. Because of the brisk circulation of CSF, 10 cc will be repleted within 30 minutes.

Specialist Consultation

Consultations are common in emergency medicine. They are not standard of care for patients with headache; however, if consultation is obtained, be clear about what the question you are asking and what clinical information you have communicated. In medico-legal cases, when there is a telephonic consult, it is not uncommon for there to be ambiguity or frank disagreements as to what was communicated to the consultant or when it was communicated. In the absence of audio recordings, it is important for the chart to be very clear about these details. Even when telemedicine is used, it is important to document whether the neurologist examined the patient via video.

Medical Decision-making, Documentation, and Communication

Based on all of the information available at this point in the care process, it is important to document your thinking in sufficient detail that someone reading the chart later will understand what you did and why. It is best to specifically document findings (or their absence) in the chart.

In depositions, physicians sometimes testify that "I only chart 'that finding' if it is positive." This is not a wise practice.

If the headache began gradually, say so. Even better, define the time that it took to reach maximal intensity (ie, the headache began around noon and gradually increased till it reached maximum intensity at 4 PM). If the temporal arteries are normal in an elderly patient, document it. Write that the neck is supple. Besides being clinically useful, this documentation helps reduce medico-legal exposure by showing your thought process and highlighting diagnostic possibilities you were considering. Although it can be difficult on a busy shift, in terms of risk management, there is no substitute for a contemporaneously written chart that spells out your concerns and thought process.

Clear communication among emergency clinicians (eg, nurses and doctors), between clinicians of different specialties (eg, neurologists or radiologists and emergency clinicians) and between clinicians and patients and families, can all prevent or mitigate medico-legal issues. One common issue is discrepant findings between the triage note and physician's history; these should be reconciled in the chart. An easy way to do this is to acknowledge the statement made in the triage note, and then to clarify it. For example, "the triage note states that the patient had a sudden onset of headache; however, when I asked the patient to clarify, they stated that it took 2 ½ hours to reach maximum intensity." This approach leaves no margin for interpretation.

Telephone discussions between consultants are potentially problematic. There is a big difference between saying "discussed with neurology" and "I told the neurologist [fill in details of the case] and she reviewed the brain imaging remotely." Unless the phone calls are recorded, it is easy for either participant to later have different recollections ("the emergency physician never told me X") since there is usually no notation in the consultant's records.

EMERGENT TREATMENTS IN THE EMERGENCY DEPARTMENT

Table 3 lists emergent time-dependent treatments to be considered for patients with headache, some of which may be started without specialist consultation and others of which may be reasonable to first discuss with the relevant consultant.

Table 3
Acute time-dependent treatments to be considered in the emergency department

Intervention	Condition
Blood pressure control	Hypertensive crisis, preeclampsia and eclampsia, PRES, SAH, ischemic, and hemorrhagic stroke
High concentration or hyperbaric oxygen	Carbon monoxide poisoning
Ocular drops to reduce intraocular pressure	Acute narrow-angle glaucoma
IV antibiotics	Bacterial meningitis, brain abscess
Steroids	Giant cell arteritis (IV if visual symptoms) or severe vasogenic edema from abscess or tumor[a]
Lumbar puncture with large volume spinal fluid removal to reduce ICP	Idiopathic intracranial hypertension
Anticoagulation reversal	Patients with ICH on anticoagulants or patients in need of an STAT procedure on an anticoagulant
Nimodipine	SAH

Abbreviations: IV, intravenous; ICH, intracranial hemorrhage; ICP, intracranial pressure; PRES, posterior reversible encephalopathy syndrome; SAH, subarachnoid hemorrhage; STAT, emergent or urgent.
[a] If CNS lymphoma is one of the possible diagnoses, usually suggested by imaging, avoid steroids when possible as a single dose of which can alter the histology and interfere with diagnosis. In the presence of severe symptomatic edema, discuss with the neurosurgical consultant but they may be necessary in some cases.

DISCHARGE CRITERIA, INSTRUCTIONS, AND AMBIGUITY

Most ED patients with headache and a normal neurologic examination are safe for discharge. Many patients with secondary causes of headache will require admission for definitive treatment. But there will be patients in the middle ground—those in whom diagnosis at the initial visit is difficult and who are discharged. In such cases, there is no substitute for sitting down, or if you are standing, consciously using body language to "be there" with the patient, and explaining that the diagnosis is not clear and that this is not uncommon in the ED. Explain what tests have been done and their significance, taking into account limitations of the tests. Give careful return instructions about what should trigger a return to the ED. Document the discussion. This simple patient-centric conversation can go a long way to avoid subsequent litigation, even in the setting of a misdiagnosis with a poor outcome.

Finally, communicating areas of ambiguity to patients and their families is an important skill for emergency physicians. Unless there is a definitive diagnosis, there is often varying degrees of diagnostic uncertainty in discharged patients. Learning to share this and having a bit of humility can be an important factor in avoiding lawsuits, even when the diagnosis turns out to be wrong.

FUTURE DIRECTIONS

Artificial intelligence for image interpretation is in its infancy and may impact sensitivity of every modality for various diagnoses going forward. Regarding optic fundus examination, deep learning,[62] iPhones,[63] and robotic optical coherence tomography[64] may all circumvent declining clinical use of fundoscopy. Templated electronic medical records that push front-line clinicians to obtain relevant information may also help with misdiagnosis.

SUMMARY

Using basic tenets of clinical medicine—accurate history-taking, targeted physical examination using a logical process to whittle down the differential diagnosis—coupled with applying the right tests when indicated, and understanding their inherent limitations, should reduce misdiagnosis. Good communication techniques and documentation should avoid or mitigate medico-legal actions when a diagnosis is missed or delayed.

CLINICS CARE POINTS

- Best practice is to mentally run through the checklist of "cannot miss" diagnoses before the patient is discharged.
- Take a careful history that includes a detailed history of present illness (HPI) and presence or absence of relevant red flags.
- Relevant elements of the history and physical examination (positive or negative) should be documented in the chart.
- Understand the limitations of diagnostic tests.
- Good communication with the patient and between members of the care team and documentation of these interactions can help reduce the likelihood of misdiagnosis or medico-legal consequences if there is one.

DISCLOSURE

The author reviews medical malpractice cases, some of which deal with acute headache, for both plaintiff and defense firms.

REFERENCES

1. Pitts SR, Niska RW, Xu J, et al. National hospital ambulatory medical care survey: 2006 emergency department summary. Natl Health Stat Report 2008;(7):1–38.
2. Lipton RB, Bigal ME, Diamond M, et al. Migraine prevalence, disease burden, and the need for preventive therapy. Neurology 2007;68(5):343–9.
3. Collaborators GBDH. Global, regional, and national burden of migraine and tension-type headache, 1990-2016: a systematic analysis for the Global Burden of Disease Study 2016. Lancet Neurol 2018;17(11):954–76.
4. Cortel-LeBlanc MA, Orr SL, Dunn M, et al. Managing and preventing migraine in the emergency department: a review. Ann Emerg Med 2023;82(6):732–51.
5. Flum DR, Morris A, Koepsell T, et al. Has misdiagnosis of appendicitis decreased over time? a population-based analysis. JAMA 2001;286(14):1748–53.
6. Grewal K, Austin PC, Kapral MK, et al. Missed strokes using computed tomography imaging in patients with vertigo: population-based cohort study. Stroke 2015; 46(1):108–13.
7. Edlow JA. Managing patients with nontraumatic, severe, rapid-onset headache. Ann Emerg Med 2018;71(3):400–8.
8. de Bruijn SF, Stam J, Kappelle LJ. Thunderclap headache as first symptom of cerebral venous sinus thrombosis. CVST Study Group. Lancet 1996;348(9042):1623–5.

9. Wasay M, Kojan S, Dai AI, et al. Headache in cerebral venous thrombosis: incidence, pattern and location in 200 consecutive patients. J Headache Pain 2010;11(2):137–9.

10. von Babo M, De Marchis GM, Sarikaya H, et al. Differences and similarities between spontaneous dissections of the internal carotid artery and the vertebral artery. Stroke 2013;44(6):1537–42.

11. Valentinis L, Tuniz F, Valent F, et al. Headache attributed to intracranial tumours: a prospective cohort study. Cephalalgia 2010;30(4):389–98.

12. Brouwer MC, Coutinho JM, van de Beek D. Clinical characteristics and outcome of brain abscess: systematic review and meta-analysis. Neurology 2014;82(9): 806–13.

13. Kim JS, Lee H. Inner ear dysfunction due to vertebrobasilar ischemic stroke. Semin Neurol 2009;29(5):534–40.

14. Do TP, Remmers A, Schytz HW, et al. Red and orange flags for secondary headaches in clinical practice: SNNOOP10 list. Neurology 2019;92(3):134–44.

15. Edjlali M, Rodriguez-Régent C, Hodel J, et al. Subarachnoid hemorrhage in ten questions. Diagn Interv Imaging 2015;96(7–8):657–66.

16. Pohl H. Red flags in headache care. Headache 2022;62(4):534–5.

17. Pohl H, Do TP, García-Azorín D, et al. Green flags and headache: a concept study using the Delphi method. Headache 2021;61(2):300–9.

18. Silberstein SD. Headaches due to nasal and paranasal sinus disease. Neurol Clin 2004;22(1):1–19.

19. Ravishankar K. Looking at "thunderclap headache" differently? Circa 2016. Ann Indian Acad Neurol 2016;19(3):295–301.

20. Perry JJ, Stiell IG, Sivilotti MLA, et al. Clinical decision rules to rule out subarachnoid hemorrhage for acute headache. JAMA 2013;310(12):1248–55.

21. Grooters GS, Sluzewski M, Tijssen CC. How often is thunderclap headache caused by the reversible cerebral vasoconstriction syndrome? Headache 2014; 54(4):732–5.

22. Kim T, Ahn S, Sohn CH, et al. Reversible cerebral vasoconstriction syndrome at the emergency department. Clin Exp Emerg Med 2015;2(4):203–9.

23. Kim WY. In: Edlow JA, editor. Personal communication - frequency of RCVS in ED patients with thunderclap headache. 2017.

24. Ducros A, Bousser MG. Thunderclap headache. BMJ 2013;346:e8557.

25. Headache Classification Committee of the International Headache Society (IHS) The International Classification of Headache Disorders, 3rd edition. Cephalalgia 2018;38(1):1–211.

26. Do TP, la Cour Karottki NF, Ashina M. Updates in the diagnostic approach of headache. Curr Pain Headache Rep 2021;25(12):80.

27. Vazquez-Barquero A, Ibáñez FJ, Herrera S, et al. Isolated headache as the presenting clinical manifestation of intracranial tumors: a prospective study. Cephalalgia 1994;14(4):270–2.

28. Shindler KS, Sankar PS, Volpe NJ, et al. Intermittent headaches as the presenting sign of subacute angle-closure glaucoma. Neurology 2005;65(5):757–8.

29. Kelly R. Colloid cysts of the third ventricle; analysis of twenty-nine cases. Brain 1951;74(1):23–65.

30. Yenermen MH, Bowerman CI, Haymaker W. Colloid cyst of the third ventricle; a clinical study of 54 cases in the light of previous publications. Acta Neuroveg 1958;17(3–4):211–77.

31. Bezuidenhout AF, Chang YM, Heilman CB, et al. Headache in Chiari Malformation. Neuroimaging Clin N Am 2019;29(2):243–53.

32. Nishijima DK, Offerman SR, Ballard DW, et al. Immediate and delayed traumatic intracranial hemorrhage in patients with head trauma and preinjury warfarin or clopidogrel use. Ann Emerg Med 2012;59(6):460–8, e1-7.
33. Edlow JA, Panagos PD, Godwin SA, et al. Clinical policy: critical issues in the evaluation and management of adult patients presenting to the emergency department with acute headache. Ann Emerg Med 2008;52(4):407–36.
34. Edlow JA, Hoffmann B. Managing patients with acute visual loss. Ann Emerg Med 2022;79(5):474–84.
35. Chan FLY, Lester S, Whittle SL, et al. The utility of ESR, CRP and platelets in the diagnosis of GCA. BMC Rheumatol 2019;3:14.
36. Edlow AG, Edlow BL, Edlow JA. Diagnosis of acute neurologic emergencies in pregnant and postpartum women. Emerg Med Clin North Am 2016;34(4):943–65.
37. Edlow JA, Caplan LR, O'Brien K, et al. Diagnosis of acute neurological emergencies in pregnant and post-partum women. Lancet Neurol 2013;12(2):175–85.
38. Greige T, Bilello LA, Singleton JM, et al. Acute headache in pregnant and postpartum patients: a clinical review. Am J Emerg Med 2023;72:16–9.
39. Schievink WI. Spontaneous intracranial hypotension. N Engl J Med 2021;385(23):2173–8.
40. Schoenen J, Sandor PS. Headache with focal neurological signs or symptoms: a complicated differential diagnosis. Lancet Neurol 2004;3(4):237–45.
41. Goldstein L, Laytman T, Steiner I. Is head computerized tomography indicated for the workup of headache in patients with intact neurological examination. Eur Neurol 2018;80(5–6):341–4.
42. Schwenkenbecher P, Pul R, Wurster U, et al. Common and uncommon neurological manifestations of neuroborreliosis leading to hospitalization. BMC Infect Dis 2017;17(1):90.
43. Krishnamoorthy A, Joel A, Abhilash KP. Cryptococcal meningitis with multiple cranial nerves palsies: a review of literature. J Global Infect Dis 2015;7(3):123–4.
44. Li X, Ma L, Zhang L, et al. Clinical characteristics of tuberculous meningitis combined with cranial nerve palsy. Clin Neurol Neurosurg 2019;184:105443.
45. Theodore WH, Gendelman S. Meningeal carcinomatosis. Arch Neurol 1981;38(11):696–9.
46. Mekinian A, Maisonobe L, Boukari L, et al. Characteristics, outcome and treatments with cranial pachymeningitis: a multicenter French retrospective study of 60 patients. Medicine (Baltim) 2018;97(30):e11413.
47. Mackay DD, Garza PS, Bruce BB, et al. The demise of direct ophthalmoscopy: a modern clinical challenge. Neurol Clin Pract 2015;5(2):150–7.
48. Kelly AM, Kuan WS, Chu KH, et al. Epidemiology, investigation, management, and outcome of headache in emergency departments (HEAD study)-a multinational observational study. Headache 2021;61(10):1539–52.
49. Kelly AM. Direct ophthalmoscopy in the evaluation of emergency department patients with headache: time to rethink? Emerg Med Australas 2023;35(2):357–8.
50. Ohle R, McIsaac SM, Woo MY, et al. Sonography of the optic nerve sheath diameter for detection of raised intracranial pressure compared to computed tomography: a systematic review and meta-analysis. J Ultrasound Med 2015;34(7):1285–94.
51. Singleton J, Dagan A, Edlow JA, et al. Real-time optic nerve sheath diameter reduction measured with bedside ultrasound after therapeutic lumbar puncture in a patient with idiopathic intracranial hypertension. Am J Emerg Med 2015;33(6):860 e5–e7.

52. Hansen HC, Helmke SS, Helmke K. Time course of optic nerve sheath dilation: in vitro response characteristics to controlled pressure elevations. J Neurol Sci 2022;441:120358.
53. Bruce BB, Lamirel C, Wright DW, et al. Nonmydriatic ocular fundus photography in the emergency department. N Engl J Med 2011;364(4):387–9.
54. Dunn HP, Teo KZ, Smyth JW, et al. Using non-mydriatic fundus photography to detect fundus pathology in Australian metropolitan emergency departments: a prospective prevalence and diagnostic accuracy study. Emerg Med Australas 2021;33(2):302–9.
55. Buyck PJ, Zuurbier SM, Garcia-Esperon C, et al. Diagnostic accuracy of noncontrast CT imaging markers in cerebral venous thrombosis. Neurology 2019;92(8): e841–51.
56. Xu W, Gao L, Li T, et al. The performance of CT versus MRI in the differential diagnosis of cerebral venous thrombosis. Thromb Haemost 2018;118(6):1067–77.
57. Kroll KE, Camacho MA, Gautam S, et al. Findings of chronic sinusitis on brain computed tomography are not associated with acute headaches. J Emerg Med 2014;46(6):753–9.
58. Edlow JA. What are the unintended consequences of changing the diagnostic paradigm for subarachnoid hemorrhage after brain computed tomography to computed tomographic angiography in place of lumbar puncture? Acad Emerg Med 2010;17(9):991–5 ; discussion 996-7.
59. Ozsvath RR, Casey SO, Lustrin ES, et al. Cerebral venography: comparison of CT and MR projection venography. AJR Am J Roentgenol 1997;169(6):1699–707.
60. Abbrescia KL, Brabson TA, Dalsey WC, et al. The effect of lower-extremity position on cerebrospinal fluid pressures. Acad Emerg Med 2001;8(1):8–12.
61. Li Y, Carandang RA, Ade S, et al. Ultrasound-guided lumbar puncture improves success rate and efficiency in overweight patients. Neurol Clin Pract 2020;10(4): 307–13.
62. Biousse V, Najjar RP, Tang Z, et al. Application of a deep learning system to detect papilledema on nonmydriatic ocular fundus photographs in an emergency department. Am J Ophthalmol 2024;261:199–207.
63. Bruce BB, Newman NJ, Biousse V. Nonmydriatic digital ocular fundus photography with iPhone 3G–reply. JAMA Ophthalmol 2013;131(3):406.
64. Song A, Roh KM, Lusk JB, et al. Robotic optical coherence tomography retinal imaging for emergency department patients: a pilot study for emergency physicians' diagnostic performance. Ann Emerg Med 2023;81(4):501–8.

Neurologic Specific Risk
Strokes, Lytics, and Litigation

Evie G. Marcolini, MD, MBE*

KEYWORDS

- Emergency medicine • Risk management • Headache • Stroke • Thrombolytics

KEY POINTS

- Take the time to get a complete and thorough history.
- Perfect and perform the neurologic examination.
- Understand the strengths and limitations of neurologic imaging.
- Be aware that there is more litigation for not giving thrombolytics for stroke.

NEUROLOGIC SPECIFIC RISK: HEADACHES AND STROKES, THROMBOLYTICS AND PITFALLS

What is the best way to avoid litigation? Take good care of the patient.
—David Stuchiner, MD.

Misdiagnosis in emergency medicine can be associated with patient harm, with neurologic diagnoses among the most common conditions to confound physicians. These are often complex, time-sensitive, and nuanced, offering opportunity for mimics and chameleons to make assessment, diagnosis, and treatment challenging. Stroke is the most common nontraumatic category associated with malpractice claims in emergency medicine,[1] in addition to spinal cord compression and injury, venous thromboembolism, meningitis, encephalitis, traumatic brain injury, traumatic intracranial hemorrhage, and spinal and intracranial abscess.

Diagnostic and treatment errors are the foundational source of malpractice litigation. While there are no data to show a direct association between errors and lawsuits in emergency medicine, the most common errors leading to harm include clinical decision-making, diagnostic assessment, and ordering and interpretation of tests.[2] Less than 2% of medically negligent care results in a malpractice claim,[3] and there is a bias toward higher severity cases.[4] In one study, neurologic cases had the highest mean payout per malpractice claim.[5]

Emergency Medicine and Neurocritical Care, Dartmouth-Hitchcock Medical Center, Lebanon, NH, USA
* Corresponding author
E-mail address: emarcolini@gmail.com

Emerg Med Clin N Am 43 (2025) 81–91
https://doi.org/10.1016/j.emc.2024.05.028
emed.theclinics.com
0733-8627/25/© 2024 Elsevier Inc. All rights are reserved, including those for text and data mining, AI training, and similar technologies.

When comparing the ratio of disability to death for disease categories, most vascular catastrophes have a 2.4 fold higher chance of death over disability, but in the case of stroke, this is reversed with a 1.9 fold higher chance of disability over death.[5] When this is figured into malpractice cases, a younger patient can be facing a longer lifespan requiring significant costly care.

Tort law is the practice of law that addresses civil wrongs, as opposed to contractual law or criminal law. Medical malpractice is a subset of tort law and is under the jurisdiction of state, as opposed to federal courts. Personal injury lawsuits include physical, emotional, or property damages caused to a person as a consequence of negligence. Fifteen percent of personal injury lawsuits involve medical malpractice, and of those that proceed to trial, 92% are decided for the defense.[6]

Emergency medicine physicians are among the most often named defendants in cases of acute stroke with the most likely reason for litigation being failure to timely diagnose (including ordering and correctly interpreting imaging) and failure to timely treat (including with thrombolytics and/or referral for thrombectomy).[7,8] In one study of 246 medical malpractice cases related to ischemic stroke, 22% of cases were based on failure to make a timely referral to a specialist, underlying the importance of consulting neurology or neurosurgery as appropriate in cases of acute stroke irrespective of a physician's planned treatment. It was alleged that 12% of patients in this study did not have timely transfer to another hospital with higher level of stroke treatment resources.[7]

Failure to Diagnose – Setting the Stage

In patients with acute ischemic stroke, diagnostic error is consistently the most common failure cited in malpractice claims. A physician may miss a diagnosis because the patient does not present with obvious signs and symptoms, such as dizziness, nausea, and vomiting in a posterior circulation stroke, or because the patient demographics are atypical to the disease, such as a young otherwise healthy person presenting with a stroke from a vertebral artery dissection. The causes of diagnostic errors in the ED are mostly rooted in the area of clinical decision-making.

A survey of claims involving patients with ischemic stroke from 2006 to 2016 found that 49.2% involved alleged diagnostic error, and approximately half of those occurred in the emergency department (ED).[8] Notably, nearly two-thirds of the ED claims analyzed involved the ongoing assessment/reassessment of patients' symptoms, a step that includes monitoring and communication of clinical changes. While much of emergency medicine training and education is directed toward history taking, physical examination, and appropriate diagnostics, these data point to reassessment and ongoing communication as key areas to improve patient safety and decrease the risk of malpractice litigation.

"Stroke chameleons" describe the false-negative cases in which acute stroke is not appropriately identified. A large, population-based study of hospitalized patients with ischemic stroke found that 14% of these chameleons were missed in the ED.[9] This number was likely an underestimate, not accounting for patients who were never correctly diagnosed and either hospitalized or discharged from the ED with the most common diagnosis being altered mental status (AMS), seen in nearly a third of the chameleons identified. While a decreased level of consciousness can confound our ability to get a detailed physical examination and can point to more generalized cerebral dysfunction secondary to a systemic illness, the neurologic examination should focus on teasing out focal or lateralizing deficits that could point to brainstem pathology.

Other symptoms that were present when a diagnosis of acute ischemic stroke was missed:

- Focal weakness
- Focal numbness
- Speech difficulty
- Headache
- Vision problems
- Dizziness/vertigo

Diagnosis Pitfalls

Specific aspects of failure to diagnose include failing to order a test, or to interpret the test correctly.[2] Patient history is key to developing a differential diagnosis, and it is important to recognize that a nonspecific neurologic complaint such as dizziness, weakness, or headache can be based in many clinical neurologic diagnoses, including anterior or posterior stroke, subarachnoid hemorrhage, posterior reversible encephalopathy syndrome (PRES), among many others. The best history taking is intentional— asking enough questions to narrow the differential appropriately, and not relying on a single simple answer from a patient who may not understand the question. For instance, asking patients what their dizziness "feels like" is not as useful as asking when it started, how long it lasts and whether anything triggers it.[10] Time spent in gathering accurate historical data including a clear understanding of end points of questions as well as a directed examination, will allow for an expanded differential that can be focused for a directed evaluation.

The importance of a full neurologic examination cannot be overstated in the setting of litigation for neurologic complaints. This component of the assessment will be dissected in every medical malpractice case and is the strongest foundation of accurate diagnostic decision-making. A common pitfall is not testing a patient's gait. Testing gait can be a sensitive indicator for pathology in the posterior fossa, which is also an anatomic area not seen very well on noncontrast computed tomography (CT) imaging. This creates 2 very common mistakes that can lead to a missed diagnosis in a condition that is very commonly missed by emergency physicians and neurologists alike.[11]

A common temptation is to order imaging based on patient complaint before a thorough history and physical examination, and this practice can lead to premature closure when the imaging does not support or is not adequately sensitive to exclude the presupposed diagnosis. Anchoring on a negative test result can be falsely reassuring to the physician as well as the patient, so it is a good practice to articulate what exactly is being evaluated with each test, and how the results will be interpreted. For instance, for a complaint of dizziness, it would be important to explain beforehand that a noncontrast head CT will rule out intracerebral hemorrhage but will not rule out posterior circulation stroke.

In patients with neurologic disease, such as stroke, imaging is in many cases a cornerstone of diagnosis, but imaging has many limitations and specificities, and there are multiple components of obtaining imaging that contribute to diagnostic error. Communication of pertinent clinical information from the ordering to the interpreting physician is paramount, not only for ordering the correct type of imaging, but also for sensitive and accurate interpretation of the images. Whether to order imaging, and which imaging to utilize, is very commonly misunderstood, and collaboration between the emergency physician and radiologist can be extremely helpful in mitigating risk.

The most commonly ordered image for patients with headache, dizziness, or neurologic weakness is a noncontrast head CT. It is very easy to order a noncontrast CT, but there are significant limitations to its sensitivity and specificity. Overreliance on noncontrast CT can result in missed diagnosis. In the case of patients with vestibular complaints, obtaining a noncontrast CT and discharging the patient home after a negative study have been associated with twice the relative risk of early stroke within 30 or 90 days compared to those who did not receive imaging at all.[12] This is likely due to a missed diagnosis of posterior circulation stroke, as the sensitivity of a noncontrast CT for ischemic changes in the posterior fossa is very low.[13] The importance of understanding what the sensitivity and specificity for noncontrast CT is for particular neurologic complaints is paramount to avoid false reassurance and/or a missed diagnosis. Other diagnoses not reliably excluded with a noncontrast brain CT include

1. Meningitis/encephalitis
2. Carbon monoxide toxicity
3. Giant cell arteritis
4. Idiopathic intracranial hypertension (pseudotumor cerebri)
5. Acute angle closure glaucoma
6. Carotid artery dissection
7. Cerebral venous thrombosis
8. Preeclampsia/eclampsia
9. PRES

Test interpretation is a common challenge in neurologic cases, as there are many imaging modalities available for the evaluation of a patient with stroke symptoms, including CT, CT angiography (CTA), CT venography (CTV), MRI, MR angiography (MRA), MR venography (MRV), and CT and MR perfusion. These imaging capabilities have advanced at a rapid pace over the last decades, and the utility and appropriate use of each one may be best determined through a collaborative conversation with either a neurologist or radiologist. While emergency medicine (EM) physicians are not expected to interpret radiologic images, it is extremely important to understand the capabilities of each test, as well as anticipated findings and their significance. In the neurologic realm, this is particularly pertinent, since there are many available imaging modalities and each one has a specific utility. One example of a pitfall of noncontrast CT is reliance on the findings to rule out a subarachnoid hemorrhage.

While noncontrast head CT has been shown to be extremely sensitive for blood in the subarachnoid space if performed within 6 hours of the onset of headache (with other requirements including a minimum third-generation CT scanner), no test is 100% sensitive or accurate. If the pretest index of suspicion is very high (significant risk factors, concerning history, etc.), it is prudent to have a conversation with the radiologist to ensure that they clearly understand the clinical picture and anticipated findings, and to consider additional testing (such as lumbar puncture) to rule out a diagnosis that can have devastating results.

This principle applies to the use of any imaging, and in all clinical settings. Know what your clinical index of suspicion is, what you expect to find from a study, and how it will be used in your decision-making. The emergency physician has the benefit of a thorough history and physical examination, and any testing including imaging should contribute to affirming or excluding the presumptive diagnosis.

Other advanced imaging modalities can be used for decision-making, such as a CT or MR perfusion for some cases of acute ischemic stroke (to determine the ratio of infarct to penumbra). However, not every neuroradiologist or neurointerventionalist is supportive of its use in clinical decision-making. The bottom line is that neuroimaging plays a significant role in decision-making, but it has multiple nuances to its use, including when to order, specifics of technologic capability, what results will show, and how they should be interpreted for clinical use. Simple reliance on the "result" of obtained imaging is fraught with the potential for misapplication, misinterpretation, and overreliance. Be careful to understand the uses and limitations of any test ordered or consult with an ancillary expert to determine its best use and/or interpretation.

Best practice

- Consider a neurologic cause in any patient with AMS.
- Perfect the complete neurologic examination.
- Do not neglect to walk the patient.
- Consider stroke in patients of any age.
- Be intentional in taking a history.
- Understand the limitations of testing, especially the commonly used noncontrast CT head.

Treatment Pitfalls

It is well worth considering the plaintiff perspective of stroke malpractice. The developments of effective therapies such as intravenous thrombolysis in 1995, subsequent advances in endovascular treatment, and advanced imaging have all presented opportunities for improved outcome for stroke in a field that prior to these developments had relatively little but supportive care for patients. These developments led to guidelines developed by the Joint Commission and AHA/ASA.[14] The Joint Commission can award certifications for acute stroke ready, primary stroke center, thrombectomy capable, or comprehensive stroke center to qualifying hospitals. The availability of effective therapeutic opportunity for a devastating disease, nationally accepted guidelines, and hospitals advertising their capabilities within that structure creates a near-perfect landscape for the proliferation of medical malpractice that has been observed over the last few decades. An aging population, consolidation of stroke systems of care, and the increasing use of tele-stroke technology will likely continue to shape what constitutes standard of care (SOC) for patients with suspected stroke. The malpractice attorney will invest significant resources to litigate the case, and with almost 800,000 strokes per year in the United States, the plaintiff will choose cases where there is a possible deviation from the abovementioned guidelines and/or an adverse outcome.[15]

Malpractice cases in acute stroke care have frequently involved thrombolytics—and more specifically, the failure to administer these medications—for nearly 3 decades. Multiple retrospective studies[16] have shown that nearly all identified cases have been associated with a failure to give or a delay in administering systemic thrombolysis, and not due to a complication (ie, hemorrhage) from administration of the thrombolytic. In fact, the risk of intracranial hemorrhage from intravenous thrombolytics in patients with acute ischemic stroke is 0.5%, and in patients with stroke mimics, it is 0.3%.[17]

In many American states, there is a requirement for a plaintiff to prove that there is a greater than 50% chance that the patient's outcome would have been better and had their condition been treated appropriately ("more likely than not" doctrine). This has historically been a challenge to cases alleging failure to administer thrombolysis, because many accepted trials show a more modest treatment effect. Mechanical thrombectomy (MT) has since been shown to have a more robust treatment effect; an odds ratio of 2.46 for reaching functional independence was cited in the HERMES meta-analysis of the 5 major trials establishing the efficacy of MT.[18] As the window for thrombectomy has widened from 6 to 24 hours in published guidelines, it is reasonable to expect growing litigation from failure to provide thrombectomy within this time frame. One study of large legal databases found 7 cases involving thrombectomy even before the pivotal studies were published in 2015 establishing the efficacy of mechanical thrombectomy.[7]

A plaintiff must show that, more likely than not, the physician did not meet the SOC, a concept that has many challenging aspects. In plain language, SOC describes what a reasonable physician would do in similar circumstances. Historically SOC was allowed to be variable depending on geography, for instance, a rural physician may not be held to the same SOC as a physician in an urban tertiary care center with many more resources and advanced diagnostic and therapeutic options. However, today SOC is based more on a national standard. In emergency medicine, the SOC for a neurologic case would be established by specialty-developed guidelines and accepted practice.[14] This becomes important and complex in the world of medical malpractice cases involving stroke, since there has been historic controversy over practices such as the utilization of systemic thrombolytic therapy.

In most cases, an expert witness will be retained to help establish SOC as defined by clinical guidelines from Emergency Medicine Professional Societies as well as Neurologic, Neurosurgical and American Heart Association guidelines.[19] This is not to say that the emergency physician will be held to the standard of a neurosurgeon, but that the accepted practice in the area of stroke would have general agreement from all stakeholders as to the SOC that should happen when an emergency physician evaluates a patient with acute ischemic stroke. In the case of thrombolytic therapy, there are multiple guidelines that attest to the SOC of thrombolytics for acute ischemic stroke within the accepted time frame from the patient's last known well time.

Diagnoses such as stroke and acute myocardial infarction are unique among others in emergency medicine in that most hospitals have accepted protocols for assessment and treatment, with time parameters. In stark contrast to other chief complaints, such as abdominal pain, stroke care through these protocols is directed based on clinical presentation and has specific associated timelines. Accurate documentation in a medical decision-making (MDM) note to justify deviation from the protocols or nationally accepted guidelines is of the greatest importance, irrespective of a physician's interpretation of the efficacy of intravenous thrombolytics or entry of a patient into the stroke protocol. It is well worth considering the national stroke center guidelines as a road map for attorneys leading to their next case.

Some examples of MDM which *may* assist if there is an adverse outcome:

- Thrombolytics are not indicated for this patient based on the fact that there was prolonged duration of symptoms with a last known well time being 48 hours ago.
- Thrombolytic medication was not indicated for this patient due to the presence of intracranial hemorrhage.
- This patient's symptoms were atypical for stroke. I consulted with the neurologist via the telemedicine portal. He agrees that this is more likely an atypical migraine and thrombolytics are not indicated. He recommended that the patient can be discharged for outpatient follow-up.

There are published literature that refute the standard of thrombolytics, and some may argue that a "respectable minority" would not utilize thrombolytics, but in practice, if this approach is being employed, then a detailed explanation should be included as to why deviation from the guidelines occurred. Documenting a very clear history and physical examination, especially a full neurologic examination, is paramount to justifying clinical decision-making in the case of a patient with symptoms and signs of stroke.

State-to-state differences in malpractice litigation may have implications in a potential lawsuit. The highest incidence of litigation is in the states of New York, California, Florida, Illinois, Pennsylvania, and Texas.[7,20] Most negligence cases require the plaintiff to show that "more likely than not" the defendant did not meet the SOC. Some states allow for negligence to be established through the "loss of chance" doctrine, which states that the defendant's actions precluded the patient from having the chance of a better outcome. For example, if a patient with acute ischemic stroke presents to the ED outside the 3 to 4.5 h window of opportunity for intravenous thrombolysis, and outside the accepted window of 6 hours for thrombectomy, there may have been an opportunity for thrombectomy if perfusion imaging had been performed showing a large penumbra and small core infarct. If the perfusion imaging was never performed, it would be impossible to prove that there was such a penumbra-to-core ratio, but not obtaining the imaging could, in some states, be litigated under the loss of chance doctrine. States can also vary as to whether they have statutory caps for damages, statute of limitations for filing a claim, standard of proof of causation, or the method of presenting expert testimony.

Best practice

- Know the national guidelines and hospital protocols.
- Justify deviation from accepted guidelines/protocols with thorough documentation.

Transfer Decision Pitfalls

Guidelines for the management of acute ischemic stroke have made strong recommendations for integrated local and regional stroke systems with clear protocols for movement of patients to centers that can potentially provide thrombolytics, mechanical thrombectomy, and specialized stroke care. The failure to transfer in a timely manner was found to be associated with a higher-than-average payout in one study,[7] suggesting that this may be an area of particular legal risk. Current stroke guidelines[19] recommend that telemedicine may be used to facilitate appropriate and rapid transfer within stroke systems.[18]

Best practice

- Understand your hospital's capabilities and transfer when appropriate.

Communication Pitfalls

In stroke litigation, allegations revolve around failure to diagnosis and failure of timely treatment. This includes a timely history, examination, testing, and interpretation of testing. Common failure points can be classified as communication pitfalls.[21] It is important to be *intentional,* in other words to have a strong sense of differential diagnosis and *intentionally* pursuing information to include or exclude important neurologic diagnoses. The key is to understand which information to pursue and which to deprioritize.

For example, a patient who states that his/her symptoms started suddenly can be *asked* what he/she means by the word "*sudden*". A patient may not clearly understand the meaning and importance of the question about sudden onset when considering headache symptoms. This requires the physician to pursue a more detailed questioning about headache onset with intentionally pointed questions. ("What were you doing when the headache started?") Very specific documentation is typically more accurate.

Best practice

- Good documentation: "The patient's headache started about 3 hours prior to arrival."
- Better documentation: "The patient's headache started at noon and gradually increased, reaching maximum intensity at 3:00 PM."

If the physician simply assumes that the onset was not sudden, he may miss a diagnosis in an atypical clinical presentation. Avoid the cognitive error of confirmation bias, characterized by selectively gathering and interpreting evidence to support a preconceived belief.

Taking more time to listen to the patient, interpret their version of the history, and appropriately apply diagnostic testing through physical examination, imaging and other tests can help to avoid the pitfalls in most ED closed malpractice claims.[8] Allowing the patient to speak without interruption is a perceived challenge for busy emergency physicians, but critical to obtain important information. After all, the physician is putting together the history. Many patients will not know which part of their history is clinically critical, so they may lead with non-discriminating or unintentionally misleading information.

Once a diagnosis is reached or excluded, referral to the appropriate service is paramount to ensuring adequate a good outcome. This includes consulting neurologists for cases with stroke presentation, or referral to a center with higher level of resources in the case of patients with pathology that cannot be treated locally.

One of the most common areas of litigation and line of questioning in a litigation deposition, testimony, or trial is regarding timing of symptoms. The window of acceptability of use for intravenous thrombolysis is well defined and accepted, making it a hard line for litigation and difficult to refute if appropriately ascertained and documented. It may take persistence and forensic questioning to determine the last known well time, but it is vitally important. The 3 h window is Food and Drug Administration (FDA) approved, and if the physician does not offer a patient thrombolysis within that window, there must be solid documentation as to the reasons, which must be consistent with accepted guidelines. The 3 to 4.5 h window is not FDA approved, but it is commonly accepted, making it the SOC, supported by guidelines.[19] Once the 4.5 h window for thrombolysis has passed, the window for thrombectomy becomes the focus. This time frame has been advancing quickly, with the development of more advanced imaging techniques such as perfusion imaging and studies showing the ability of specific MRI techniques such as diffusion weighted imaging (DWI) and fluid attenuated inversion recovery (FLAIR) comparisons to determine the likely success of thrombectomy. The emergency physician is not expected to be able to apply these imaging techniques in order to determine whether a patient should be offered thrombectomy but is absolutely expected to consult a neurologic or neurosurgical expert who can.

Communication with the patient and/or surrogate is vitally important. In many cases, it will take more time to ensure that the patient understands the situation, pathology, and choices. Shared decision-making is an appropriate tool, but it must be clear to all and well documented that the patient understands the options, potential side effects of treatment and consequences of declining treatment. The additional time taken will be paramount in understanding the patient's risk-taking propensity and making certain that the choices are appropriately matched to the patient's values and goals of care, irrespective of physician opinions of the literature.

Documentation Pitfalls

The litigation process relies on what is documented by the physician and all ancillary staff associated with the patient's care. It also relies on the documented timing of actions, ordering and results of laboratories, imaging, and consultations. This cannot be overemphasized, and yet it comes home to roost in many malpractice cases. If documentation does not tell the story, a jury is left to the influence of litigating attorneys to help derive the story of what actually happened. Physicians naturally are not trained in the art and strategy of litigation, so even if they know what happened in the clinical realm, if it was not documented, a skillful attorney may characterize the lack of documentation as lack of action, or even lack of consideration.

Nowhere does this become more evident than in the documentation of the neurologic examination, including repeat examinations. One of the most common pitfalls is not performing and documenting ongoing assessment, including neurologic examination.[8] If a patient has a complaint of dizziness, and the neurologic examination is documented as "intact" but there is no documentation of the patient having been tested for a normal gait, this increases the risk of litigation should the patient ultimately be diagnosed with a posterior circulation stroke. In deposition, the patient will likely remember clearly whether he was asked to walk or not, as will his accompanying family.

Best practice

- Clearly document assessment, decision-making, and timing.
- Be aware of documentation in the chart, such as triage and/or consultant notes.
- Avoid indiscriminate use of templated charting, and do not document something that was not done.

Tele-stroke Pitfalls

Tele-stroke capabilities are a significant resource for those working in hospitals without the luxury of in-house neurology consultation. The ability to have a neurologist assess patients without having to transfer them across a geographic distance can facilitate more rapid diagnosis and treatment of time-sensitive diagnoses including acute ischemic stroke and other neurologic conditions.

In times of overcrowding and resource shortage, a tele-neurologist may provide a diagnosis and recommend therapy, but not be able to accept the patient in transfer. For example, the stroke neurologist may recommend administering thrombolytics for an acute ischemic stroke but would decline the patient for transfer to their center for thrombectomy. This leaves the referring physician with the responsibility of finding a center that will take the patient and provide thrombectomy. If the physician requesting a consult is not comfortable with a recommendation, it will be important to clarify and agree upon a treatment plan, as both physicians are vulnerable to liability if a lawsuit occurs, but the tele-physician is likely to have less liability in the end simply because he has restricted abilities to assess, and a jury is more likely to assign responsibility to the physician with the closest proximity.

The referring physician is responsible to provide all the available information, since he has the proximity and a more exhaustive ability to obtain information and examine the patient. This places more legal culpability on the physician next to the patient.

Neurologic diseases are a unique entity in the world of medical malpractice for a few reasons. The existence of specific society-approved protocols sets the stage for a relatively clear SOC, and thus a clean target for litigation. Time-sensitive and complex decision-making that requires collaboration with multiple specialties (emergency medicine, neurology, radiology) makes the care more complex. Missed diagnoses can happen in young patients, portending a loss of opportunity over a long period of time. Physician practice should not be driven by legal or malpractice considerations, but awareness of the pitfalls and best practice in this area will help to avoid litigation and improve both practice and patient outcome.

Best Practice Recommendations

- Take the time to get a complete and thorough history.
- Perfect and perform the neurologic examination.
- Understand the strengths and limitations of neurologic imaging.
- Know and follow guidelines, or explain deviation from them.
- Practice thorough and accurate documentation.
- Collaborate with and involve pertinent consultants, such as neurology and neuroradiology.
- Communicate with the patient and/or surrogate the benefits and risks of all choices.

CLINICS CARE POINTS

- Know and follow guidelines, or explain deviation from them.
- Practice thorough and accurate documentation.
- Collaborate with and involve pertinent consultants, such as neurology and neuroradiology.
- Communicate with the patient and/or surrogate the benefits and risks of all choices.

DISCLOSURE

The authors have nothing to disclose.

REFERENCES

1. Newman-Toker DE, Peterson SM, Badihian S, et al. Diagnostic errors in the emergency department: a systematic review [Internet]. Rockville (MD): Agency for Healthcare Research and Quality (US); 2022. p. 15, 18, 21. Report No: 22(23)-EHC043.
2. Ferguson B, Geralds J, Petrey J, et al. Malpractice in emergency medicine-a review of risk and mitigation practices for the emergency medicine provider. J Emerg Med 2018;55(5):659–65.
3. Localio AR, Lawthers AG, Brennan TA, et al. Relation between malpractice claims and adverse events due to negligence. results of the harvard medical practice study III. N Engl J Med 1991;325(4):245–51.
4. Studdert DM, Mello MM, Gawande AA, et al. Claims, errors, and compensation payments in medical malpractice litigation. N Engl J Med 2006;354(19): 2024–33.
5. Newman-Toker DE, Schaffer AC, Yu-Moe CW, et al. Serious misdiagnosis-related harms in malpractice claims: The "Big Three" - vascular events, infections, and cancers. Diagnosis (Berl) 2019;6(3):227–40. Erratum in: Diagnosis (Berl). 2020 May 16;8(1):127-128.
6. Wong KE, Parikh PD, Miller KC, et al. Emergency department and urgent care medical malpractice claims 2001-15. West J Emerg Med 2021;22(2):333–8.

7. Haslett JJ, Genadry L, Zhang X, et al. Systematic review of malpractice litigation in the diagnosis and treatment of acute stroke. Stroke 2019;50(10):2858–64.

8. Liberman AL, Skillings J, Greenberg P, et al. Breakdowns in the initial patient-provider encounter are a frequent source of diagnostic error among ischemic stroke cases included in a large medical malpractice claims database. Diagnosis (Berl) 2020;7(1):37–43.

9. Madsen TE, Khoury J, Cadena R, et al. Potentially missed diagnosis of ischemic stroke in the emergency department in the greater cincinnati/northern kentucky stroke study. Acad Emerg Med 2016;23(10):1128–35.

10. Newman-Toker DE, Edlow JA. TiTrATE: a novel, evidence-based approach to diagnosing acute dizziness and vertigo. Neurol Clin 2015;33(3). 577-599, viii.

11. Arch AE, Weisman DC, Coca S, et al. Missed ischemic stroke diagnosis in the emergency department by emergency medicine and neurology services. Stroke 2016;47(3):668–73. Epub 2016 Feb 4. Erratum in: Stroke. 2016 Mar;47(3):e59.

12. Grewal K, Austin PC, Kapral MK, et al. Missed strokes using computed tomography imaging in patients with vertigo: population-based cohort study. Stroke 2015; 46(1):108–13.

13. Chalela JA, Kidwell CS, Nentwich LM, et al. Magnetic resonance imaging and computed tomography in emergency assessment of patients with suspected acute stroke: a prospective comparison. Lancet 2007;369(9558):293–8.

14. Kleindorfer DO, Towfighi A, Chaturvedi S, et al. 2021 guideline for the prevention of stroke in patients with stroke and transient ischemic attack: a guideline from the american heart association/american stroke association. Stroke 2021;52(7): e364–467.

15. Tsao CW, Aday AW, Almarzooq ZI, et al, American Heart Association Council on Epidemiology and Prevention Statistics Committee and Stroke Statistics Subcommittee. Heart disease and stroke statistics-2023 update: a report from the american heart association. Circulation 2023;147(8):e93–621.

16. Ganti L, Kwon B, George A, et al. Tissue plasminogen activator and patients with acute ischemic stroke: the litigation landscape. J Am Coll Emerg Physicians Open 2022;3(1):e12646.

17. Tsivgoulis G, Zand R, Katsanos AH, et al. Safety of intravenous thrombolysis in stroke mimics: prospective 5-year study and comprehensive meta-analysis. Stroke 2015;46(5):1281–7.

18. Goyal M, Menon BK, van Zwam WH, et al. Endovascular thrombectomy after large-vessel ischaemic stroke: a meta-analysis of individual patient data from five randomised trials. Lancet 2016;387(10029):1723–31.

19. Powers WJ, Rabinstein AA, Ackerson T, et al. Guidelines for the early management of patients with acute ischemic stroke: 2019 update to the 2018 guidelines for the early management of acute ischemic stroke: a guideline for healthcare professionals from the american heart association/american stroke association. Stroke 2019;50(12):e344–418.

20. Pecorari IL, Flaquer I, Bergemann R, et al. Medical malpractice and intracranial hemorrhages in the U.S.: an analysis of 121 cases over 35 years. Heliyon 2023; 9(4):e14885.

21. Kachalia A, Gandhi TK, Puopolo AL, et al. Missed and delayed diagnoses in the emergency department: a study of closed malpractice claims from 4 liability insurers. Ann Emerg Med 2007;49(2):196–205.

Abdominal Pain-Specific Legal Risk

Andrew Kendle, MD[a],*, Colin Kaide, MD[b]

KEYWORDS

- Abdominal pain • Risk • Malpractice • Misdiagnosis • Delay • Lawsuit

KEY POINTS

- Abdominal pain is a frequent emergency department (ED complaint, is often unclear in etiology, and demonstrates perhaps the highest rate of bouncebacks and misdiagnosis.
- It is critical to know the limitations of diagnostic testing, especially abdominal imaging.
- Areas of highest risk are time-sensitive surgical diagnoses, extra-abdominal sources of pain, and special populations.
- Documentation of medical decision-making and return precautions are extremely important when diagnoses are complicated or unclear.

INTRODUCTION

Structures in the adjacent compartments (thorax, pelvis, and retroperitoneal space) can present as pain sensed in the abdomen. And due to limited, arborized innervation of the viscera that leads to poorly localized pain, intra-abdominal surgical emergencies may present as referred pain (shoulder, thorax, neck, pelvis, and scrotum).[1] These factors can lead to errors in diagnosis that can result in misses and delays in definitive care. A recent review of closed medical malpractice cases spanning from 1975 to 2007 showed the percentage of emergency medicine provider litigation attributable to abdominal pain or appendicitis was 5.7%. Cases attributable to aortic aneurysm comprised 1.9% (**Box 1**).[2]

We have come a long way since the first edition of Cope's Diagnosis of the Acute Abdomen, published in 1921[3] with many advances in diagnostic testing and imaging. Despite ultrasound, computed tomography (CT), and MRI, the prudent emergency physician (EP) must still be aware of the limitations of diagnostic testing and heed the

a Department of Emergency Medicine at the University of California at San Francisco Medical Center, 521 Parnassus Avenue, San Francisco, CA 94143, USA; b Department of Emergency Medicine at the Ohio State University, 776 Prior Hall, 376 West 10th Avenue, Columbus, OH 43210, USA
* Corresponding author.
E-mail address: p_kendle@yahoo.com

Emerg Med Clin N Am 43 (2025) 93–113
https://doi.org/10.1016/j.emc.2024.05.027
emed.theclinics.com
0733-8627/25/© 2024 Elsevier Inc. All rights are reserved, including those for text and data mining, AI training, and similar technologies.

> **Box 1**
> **Pattern recognition for bariatric complications**
>
> History of bariatric surgery with
> 1. New acute abdominal pain.
> 2. New vague abdominal pain in association with unexplained tachycardia and dyspnea.
> 3. New acute intermittent abdominal pain.
> 4. Signs and symptoms of bowel obstruction.
> 5. Signs and symptoms of peritonitis.

teachings of Zachary Cope, now in its 22nd edition, of the importance of experience and clinical observation based on careful history taking and physical examination[4]:

All who have had much experience of the group of cases known generally as the acute abdomen will probably agree that in that condition early diagnosis is exceptional. There are still many who do not appreciate to the full significance of the earlier and less flagrant symptoms of acute abdominal disease
                                                      —*Preface, 1st Edition.*

ANATOMY OF A LAWSUIT

A physician (or nonphysician provider) is held to the "standard of care." This definition has evolved over the years but in its most common form is "That which a minimally competent physician in the same field would do under similar circumstances."[5–8]

Medical–legal risk usually stems from 1 of 3 situations:

- Failure to make the correct diagnosis.
- Failure to make the diagnosis in a timely manner.
- Failure to initiate treatment in a timely manner.

In a legal sense, when factual information is not known to a physician but it is within his or her scope of practice to know this information, the error may be categorized as a "knew or should have known!" situation, leaving the clinician open to liability. It is best to avoid this by staying on top of one's game and being prepared for the causes of disease or pain in their various incarnations overall populations of patients one is responsible for.

SCOPE OF THIS STUDY

This article first focuses on a few of the more common diagnoses that present as abdominal pain and have been shown to be sources of litigation, largely due to misdiagnosis or delay in treatment. The authors explore the presentation, pitfalls, and pearls for the diagnosis of these problems. The authors then present problems that appear in the bariatric population because these have been less frequently addressed in our literature.

IMAGING CHARACTERISTICS: YOUR TESTS CAN LIE TO YOU

Advances in imaging are presumed to have significantly lowered the incidence of missed or severely delayed diagnosis in abdominal pain, though literature lags behind practice. However, misdiagnosis is still quite common, as abdominal pain carries a broad differential diagnosis with a high rate of benign etiologies and recurrent presentations.[9] Thus, it is key for the practitioner to understand the limitations of testing.

Cited sensitivities are listed in **Table 1**. As a general rule, diagnostic performance of imaging to rule out emergent surgical pathology is insufficient in cases of high clinical suspicion. Notably, in the Cochrane review for appendicitis, at a moderately high

Table 1
Sensitivities of typical venous phase contrast-enhanced computed tomography and ultrasound imaging for various abdominal processes

	CT Abdomen	Ultrasound
Appendicitis[10,12–16]	95% (non-contrast 92.7%)	40%–95%
Cholecystitis[17,18]	85%	68%–81%
Gallstones[19]	75%	96%
Acute Mesenteric Ischemia[20,21]	83%	85%
Ovarian Torsion[22]	74%–95%	80%

pretest probability of 40%, the authors note that following a negative CT, the posttest probability of appendicitis remains 4%.[10] CT angiogram (CTA) for mesenteric ischemia is only 90% sensitive.[11] Investigations for ovarian torsion are even worse.[1] In short, your tests can lie to you, and in cases of high clinical suspicion, consultation may be required even with normal imaging. In addition to the clinician understanding the limitations of testing, it is important that the patient knows that a normal image does not mean "nothing is wrong" and will come back if their pain worsens, changes, or does not resolve; studies suggest that good return precautions are critical even for those with CT imaging, as new or worsening diagnoses are common.[11] It is also prudent to build pathways or systems of care for diagnoses such as cholecystitis, ectopic pregnancy, and ovarian torsion that most frequently evade our imaging.

THE IMPORTANCE OF COMMUNICATION

Bouncebacks! And follow-up. Abdominal pain has one of the highest rates of bouncebacks and changes in diagnosis. Varied estimates demonstrate a rate over 20% of change in diagnosis, even as early as at 30 h scheduled return visits in nonspecific abdominal pain.[23] Extra attention should be paid to return precautions and follow-up plans as well as informing patients and documenting when follow-up for possible malignancy.

INTRA-ABDOMINAL PROCESSES
Appendicitis

Common things being common, appendicitis remains the most cited medicolegal risk among malpractice claims that are brought due to abdominal pain.[2] While this is reviewed in depth with respect to pediatrics in this issue within the study—Medical malpractice epidemiology—Adults and pediatrics by Kelly Wong Heidepriem, it is certainly an area of importance in adults as well. A review of insurance claims data demonstrated increased misdiagnosis of appendicitis in female patients, patients with comorbidities, older patients, and patients with constipation.[24]

Pearls and Perils

- *Atypical and early presentations*. When patients present with nonspecific, nonlocalized pain, or when classic symptoms such as anorexia, vomiting, or fever are absent, the diagnosis of appendicitis can be missed or delayed. This is especially true early in the course of symptoms. The most important factor to mitigate this when imaging is not obtained is to document the details of the decision-making process and to clearly instruct the patient to return for a recheck in 12 to 24 hours if the pain is not improved or becomes worse.

- *Address concerns.* Failing to discuss the risks and benefits of CT when a patient is specifically concerned about appendicitis, or failure to elicit this concern, is high risk.
- *Avoid reliance on scoring systems.* The Alvarado score has demonstrated poor sensitivity in adults and American College of Emergency Physicians (ACEP) has recommended against its use in adults in 2023.[25,26]
- *Expeditious care.* As the most common abdominal source of litigation,[27] appendicitis is an example of how delay in therapy for a correctly made diagnosis can result in malpractice suits. Clearly timed documentation of discussions with consultants and with facilities to which patients may be transferred can be protective to the EP if delays are clearly outside of our control.

Biliary Disease

Simple biliary colic does not lend itself to a high medical–legal risk. Problems involving the gallbladder arise when more complicated disease is missed because of vague localization or absence of classic findings such as Murphy's sign, elevated white blood cell (WBC) count, and fever.

- *Cholecystitis* is of increased interest due to the lack of a single definitive imaging test—ultrasound is only 68% to 80% sensitive.[17,18] However, the advantage of ultrasound in detecting gallstones is quite important. As for examination findings, fever is only 30% to 60% sensitive and right upper quadrant tenderness is the most important single finding at 96% sensitive.[28] CT scanning can be useful in the undifferentiated abdomen and is more sensitive than ultrasound for the diagnosis of acute cholecystitis.[17,29] Reliance on a single test can be deceptive; the clinician should correlate test findings with clinical findings. Of note, the hepatobiliary iminodiacetic acid (HIDA) nuclear scintigraphy scan is the noninvasive gold standard with a sensitivity still of 96%.[18]
- *Use a guideline.* The CT and/or ultrasound should be complementary and the choice for their use should depend on the diagnosis of highest consideration based on the clinical assessment. Standardize whether a nuclear scan, transfer, or consultation is the best next step.

Mesenteric Ischemia

As in the other surgical pathologies, facilitating timely surgical evaluation and management is as important as diagnosis in the reduction of medicolegal risk.

- *Back to basics.* Clinical history and examination, especially pain out of proportion and increasing age beyond 60 years (**Fig. 1**), are important pretest considerations as no test, no single finding, and not even imaging are sufficiently sensitive.[30]
- While embolic arterial mesenteric ischemia is the most common due to atrial fibrillation, remain vigilant for the more subacute or varied presenting history for thrombotic in those with vascular disease, venous in those with venous thromboembolic risk factors, and to a lesser degree nonocclusive mesenteric ischemia.[31]

PELVIC PROCESSES

Although the EP is well versed in the risk associated with pelvic sources of pain, they remain challenging diagnoses with a high element of risk, especially as we grapple with gender disparities in treatment and possible trends in pregnancy outcomes.[32–35] It is a concern that increasing public awareness of these disparities, if not addressed,

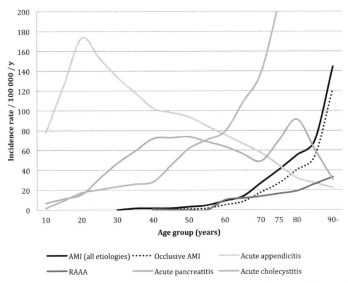

Fig. 1. Clinical history and examination, especially pain out of proportion and critically increasing age beyond 60 years.

could increase the likelihood of antagonistic encounters and litigation. The most relevant of these causes of pelvic pain to medicolegal risk are ectopic pregnancy, ovarian torsion, and pelvic inflammatory disease.

Ectopic Pregnancy

Failure to consider ectopic pregnancy should not happen as it is rare to not send a pregnancy test in a childbearing-age female individual with pelvic pain and/or bleeding. Areas of risk could be at the extremes of childbearing age, especially pediatrics, or with transgender patients.

- *Nonspecific findings.* As with mesenteric ischemia and others, no element of the history or examination is highly sensitive or specific for ectopic pregnancy.[36] Cervical motion tenderness and adnexal mass were relatively specific (positive LR 4.9, 2.4, respectively), but only transvaginal ultrasound (negative LR 0.12) was highly sensitive. This, still, is imperfect, and the true gold standard for diagnosis of ectopic is likely serial quantitative beta-human chorionic gonadotrophin (HCG) in concert with obstetrics and gynecology, which is best supported through guidelines and policy.[37,38]

Ovarian Torsion

Ovarian Torsion
  Ovarian torsion is another classically difficult diagnosis in which up to 30% of patients present without pain and no characteristic or imaging test is sufficient to rule out the diagnosis.[22,39]
  Shared decision-making with patients regarding transvaginal ultrasound and collaboration with obstetrics and gynecology colleagues are critical, especially in high-risk patients. Documentation of the conversation regarding diagnostic uncertainty and/or return precautions is a vital step.

- *Special populations.* Keep torsion in mind for pregnant and pediatric patients—in 3 case series, 12% occurred in pregnant and 15% in pediatric patients.[40–42]
- *Use caution with classic teachings.* Do not lose urgency due to ovarian size or duration of symptoms—while more common with ovarian cysts at 4 to 5 cm, torsion has been documented in cysts from 1 to 30 cm and salvage has been documented as far out as 36 hours.[39,43]
- *Imaging pitfall.* Although ultrasound with Doppler flow studies is the test of choice to evaluate for torsion, normal flow can be seen in 25% to 50% of confirmed torsion. Further, if torsion is intermittent, blood flow can appear normal at the time of Doppler studies, yet the ovary can still be in jeopardy. Combining multiple sonographic findings, ultrasound with Doppler is up to 84% sensitive for torsion.[44]

Pelvic Inflammatory Disease

Pelvic inflammatory disease (PID) is a fertility-threatening process for which no single factor is sufficiently sensitive, and a low threshold to treat is recommended for the combination of pelvic organ tenderness and inflammatory signs.[45]

It is not a difficult diagnosis when the patient presents with pelvic pain and vaginal discharge, but misdiagnosis can occur in a sexually active woman who presents with generalized abdominal pain or right upper quadrant (RUQ) pain (Fitz-Hugh–Curtis syndrome). Additionally, patients who were recently tested for the usual sexually transmitted infection (STIs) and represent with the right story could have an unusual pathogen causing unsuspected PID. *Mycoplasma genitalium* causes nongonococcal urethritis in men and PID in women. It does not grow in routine cultures and the first Food and Drug Administration-approved test appeared in 2019. Drug resistance to azithromycin is now common.[46]

- *Low threshold to treat.* Do not rule out with STI testing or lack of vaginal discharge. The latest guidelines recommend empiric PID treatment of any sexually active female patient with otherwise unexplained cervical motion, uterine *or* adnexal tenderness.[45]

EXTRAABDOMINAL PROCESSES (PAIN THAT ORIGINATES OUTSIDE OF THE ABDOMEN BUT CAN BE PERCEIVED AS ABDOMINAL PAIN)

A review of missed diagnoses shows that 43% of abdominal pain misses were extra-abdominal processes.[9] The poorly localizing sensation of the viscera can often lead to abdominal discomfort as the presenting feature of pathology outside of the abdominal cavity. This is of greatest risk in the settings of supradiaphragmatic etiologies (such as cardiac or pulmonary), the retroperitoneal vasculature, and testicular torsion.

Thoracic

Pain from inferior wall myocardial infarction (MI) may be perceived as upper abdominal/epigastric pain. When coupled with nausea and the description of "heartburn," a clinician can misdirect focus on an abdominal cause of the pain. This may be especially true when the patient is younger or female and is perceived to be of a lower risk for cardiac disease.

Pulmonary embolism has been reported to manifest solely as upper abdominal pain.[47] Similarly, pneumonias both from traditional bacterial sources and from COVID-19 can present initially with abdominal pain or discomfort. This seems to be more common in pediatric patients.[48]

When diagnostic endeavors are not fruitful in patients with upper abdominal pain that abuts the thorax, additional consideration should be given to other possible causes, including cardiac and pulmonary sources. This does not necessitate an exhaustive search in all cases but rather prudent considerations of subtle additional pieces of historical or examination data that may have been overlooked during the first pass at diagnosis.

Retroperitoneal Hematoma

Owing to the lack of symptoms and localizing signs, bleeding into the retroperitoneal space often goes unrecognized until the volume of blood loss produces systemic symptoms including overt hemorrhagic shock.[49] Retroperitoneal hematomas result from injury to parenchyma or vascular structures and can be traumatic or nontraumatic. Traumatic hematomas can result from blunt or penetrating trauma. These are much easier to find given the potential imaging that would occur in the setting of trauma significant enough to cause pelvic fractures. Blunt injuries to the pancreas can also lead to retroperitoneal hematomas amenable to visualization on CT scanning.

Nontraumatic hematomas may be harder to discover early as they are usually unanticipated. The exception is with iatrogenic cases resulting from percutaneous procedures (PCI) involving catheterization of the femoral vessels. While the mortality for retroperitoneal hematomas caused by this procedure remains significant, the incidence has been on the decline, occurring in about 0.06% of cases.[50] Unexplained blood loss, hypotension, or back pain in patients with a recent groin access procedure should undergo CT scanning to evaluate for possible retroperitoneal hematoma. Spontaneous retroperitoneal hematomas are rare but seem to occur more frequently in patients on anticoagulation.[51]

The addition of contrast to the CT is not necessary to see the hematoma but may show active extravasation and point to ongoing sites of bleeding. Focused assessment with sonography in trauma (FAST) scans are useful for the detection of intraperitoneal blood but are insensitive for retroperitoneal hematomas.[52] Trauma patients with unexpected hypotension or a drop in hemoglobin with a negative FAST scan should undergo CT imaging.

The Aorta

There are few diagnoses in emergency medicine for which both a delay in diagnosis and delay in definitive treatment have such a profound impact on outcome. Despite the ready availability of bedside ultrasound (US) and CTA of the aorta, missed aortic pathology including ruptured abdominal aortic aneurysm (AAA) and aortic dissection (AD) remains the boogeymen of our profession. Fortunately, only a small percentage of AAA and AD cases (0.01%) go on to litigation for missed diagnoses or delay of care. EPs lead the list of defendants at 29%, followed by cardiology (20%) with vascular and cardiothoracic surgery bringing up the rear at 10%.[53]

A review of the literature including classic papers such as International Registry of Acute Aortic Dissection published in JAMA in 2000 has shown us that the "classic" signs and symptoms of AD do not occur regularly and are often absent in proven cases.[54] Likewise, AAA often develop asymptomatically and show themselves only during rapid expansion or at the time of rupture.[55,56] A study looking at cases of AAA showed a 42% miss rate at initial diagnosis.[57] Further confusing the picture, classic signs of peritonitis will be absent in patients with a ruptured AAA as long as it is contained in the retroperitoneal space.

The question of greatest importance is *why do we miss these cases*? When the patient presents with the classic (or near classic) presentation of AAA or AD, imaging is almost always obtained and the diagnosis is made. But when the presentation is not classic or suggests a reasonable alternative pathology, the risk of misdiagnosis increases significantly. One meta-analysis showed that AAA presents with abdominal pain in only 61% of cases.[57] A more recent study looking specifically at cases that resulted in malpractice litigation showed similar numbers, with abdominal pain as a presenting complaint in only 52%. Similarly, back pain and/or pain radiating to the back occurred in 37%. AD also manifested as abdominal pain in 15% of cases and had back pain (or radiating to the back) in 17%. A diagnosis involving the gastrointestinal (GI) tract and genitourinary (GU) tract (nephrolithiasis) tops the list as misdiagnoses in cases of proven ruptured AAA.[53]

An additional problem that EPs face is that we are unable to provide definitive surgical care for AAA and AD; we are at the mercy of the systems in which we work. As with other time-sensitive conditions, active advocacy for the patient that is well documented is critical in protecting the EP in the case of a delay in definitive management.

It is prudent for the clinician to address patients with nonspecific presentations and at risk for cardiovascular disease to consider the question "why *does not* this patient have an aortic problem?" This does not mean that every patient needs a screening CT scan. It does mean that one should be diligent in obtaining adequate data (history and examination and assessment of pretest risk) to assure that the final diagnosis is consistent with the patient's presentation.

The Kidneys

While renal colic may be a clinical diagnosis in certain patient populations, in older patients or those in whom there is any diagnostic uncertainty, a CT of the abdomen and pelvis using a renal stone protocol should be performed. Classically, the CT scan is done without contrast to facilitate visualization of stone. Some newer CT scanners can digitally subtract administered contrast to allow for both a contrast-enhanced and a non-contrast assessment. The enhancement with contrast can allow for alternative diagnoses to be occasionally discovered.

One important consideration in ureterolithiasis is the completely obstructed ureter in the face of infection, specifically pyelonephritis. The mortality without decompression of the infected kidney approaches 20%.[58] Urology and/or interventional radiology should be consulted early for patients with ureterolithiasis with obstruction who are febrile or have other symptoms suggestive of sepsis. A high index of suspicion for infected stone should be maintained for worsening urosepsis, severe pain with urinary tract infection (UTI), or a history of nephrolithiasis.

Testicular Torsion

Testicular torsion occurs at the rate of 3.8/100,000 patient years with loss of a testicle occurring in 32% to 42% of cases.[59] Litigation in cases of missed diagnosis leading to delay in treatment is common, with torsion being among the top 4 reasons for malpractice cases in the pediatric population. In one study looking at lawsuits between 1985 and 2015 (n = 35), EPs topped the list as the defendants in 35% of cases.[59] When the data in this retrospective study and others were analyzed, a few themes arose as factors associated with litigation.

- *Atypical presentation.* We classically think of testicular torsion as presenting with relatively sudden onset of testicular pain, scrotal swelling, and tenderness. In the cases that went to litigation, testicular pain was the first presenting symptom only about half the time, with isolated abdominal pain occurring in about 30% of the cases. Other studies have shown abdominal pain as the presenting symptoms in 22% of pediatric patients.[60] These patients took longer to arrive at the diagnosis of torsion and to initiate surgical management. The physician's diagnosis was epididymitis in half of the missed cases.

- *Testicular ultrasound.* Although testicular ultrasound with color flow Doppler is considered the "gold standard" for ruling out torsion, it is imperfect. Further, an ultrasound showing flow to the testicle in question may be falsely negative in as high as 1% of cases, an approximate 89% to 95% sensitivity and 98% to 100% specificity.[61,62]
- *Timely consultation with urology.* If identified and fixed within 6 hours of onset, the salvage rate for torsion can range from 85% to 97%.[63] The urologist should be contacted immediately if torsion is suspected, that is, before test results have returned. Although the EP may get pushback from urology if the ultrasound is not yet done when contact is made, this should not dissuade the EP. Many factors can delay definitive care. First, patients may delay coming in to be seen owing to embarrassment about discussing pain in their genital region. Second, they may not present directly to an ED where testing and treatment are most likely to happen, instead going to a primary doctor's office or to an urgent care where ultrasound may not be available. Next, if they present to a non-ED setting, there is a finite amount of time that it takes to be either transferred or for the patient to get themselves to the referral hospital. Additionally, there is turn-around time to get an ultrasound, especially if the tech is not in house. Finally, there may be delays in contacting and mobilizing the urologist. It is a good practice and likely legally protective to document the times at which all of the links in the chain of care occur.
- *Failure to do a testicular examination in patients with abdominal pain.* In a number of studies looking at missed torsion, patients presenting with abdominal pain that ultimately turned out to be torsion did not have a testicular examination done. Looking specifically at cases that went to litigation, 19% did not have an examination of the testicles performed in the initial evaluation.[59]

SPECIAL POPULATIONS
Geriatric Patients

It is not surprising news that older patients may present atypically and have higher rates of pathology. This is certainly a group to have a low threshold to image; specifically keep in mind cholecystitis and mesenteric ischemia (see **Fig. 1**).

- *Misdiagnosis and examination.* Older patients are more likely to be misdiagnosed at index visit at a rate as high as 50%, have higher mortality, and are less likely to have rebound tenderness or rigidity with peritonitis.[64]
- *Anorexia.* Of special note is the association of subtle symptoms such as anorexia with mortality in presentations for abdominal pain.[65] These should prompt consideration of an expanded differential and evaluation.

A couple of good quotes have been thrown around by attending physicians in our training program, 2 of which sum up the geriatric abdomen succinctly! The first is "the machinations of elderly bellies are limitless" and second "I have rarely met an old belly I have not scanned!"

Bariatric Surgery Patients

Bariatric surgery, more formally known as "Metabolic and Bariatric Surgery," is becoming common worldwide. In the United States, more than 250,000 bariatric procedures are performed annually, making it one of the most popular elective general surgical procedures.[66] There are 4 bariatric procedures that have been traditionally

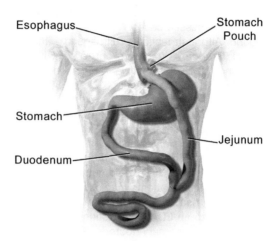

Fig. 2. Roux-en Y.

performed, with 2 being most common currently. The procedures common proced-ures include Roux-en Y (RY) and sleeve gastrectomy (SG). The adjustable gastric band (AGB) is much less commonly performed today, but patients who have had the procedure in the past can present with late complications[67] (**Figs. 2–5**).

Patients who have had bariatric surgery can present to the emergency department with complaints of abdominal pain. Because of the unique anatomy created by the surgery, certain bariatric procedures are predisposed to potentially serious complica-tions. The EP should seek out the surgeon who performed the procedure or discuss the case with a surgeon who is familiar with bariatric surgical procedures and manage-ment of their complications.

When evaluating a patient with abdominal pain who has had a bariatric procedure performed, the following information should be elicited as it will help in narrowing the differential diagnosis and aid in communication with the consulting surgeon.

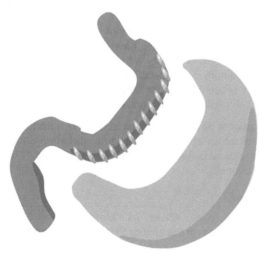

Fig. 3. Sleeve gastrectomy.

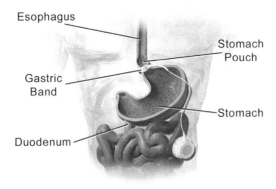

Fig. 4. Adjustable gastric banding.

- What specific procedure was performed: RY, gastric sleeve, AGB or an older, less common procedure such as a biliopancreatic diversion with duodenal switch or vertical banded gastrofundoplasty.
- When was the procedure done?
- Who did the surgery and where was it done?
- Were there any complications during the hospital stay?
- Is the pain constant or intermittent?
- Are there associated symptoms such as tachycardia, tachypnea, nausea and vomiting, fever, referred pain, or pain with movement?

Specific complications are discussed later.

Anastomotic leak
The most common early complication with any of these surgical procedures aside from infection is an anastomotic leak. In a review of bariatric surgery malpractice claims from 2017, 70% of claims were for RY patients and the most common complaint was delay in diagnosis of anastomotic leak.[68] The usual leak site is at the staple lines in RY and gastric sleeve procedures. Even though the AGB does not

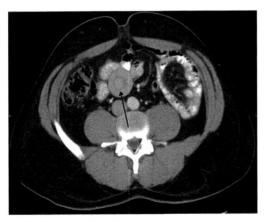

Fig. 5. "Target sign" of telescoping bowel in intussusception.

involve a cutting of gastrointestinal structures, direct injuries to the esophagus or stomach and early or late erosions of the band itself can produce leaks.[67] Signs and symptoms of an anastomotic leak are pain with signs of peritonitis and eventually the development of a fever and leukocytosis. Unexplained tachycardia and shortness of breath are nonspecific signs that may be present before the diagnosis becomes apparent.

The mortality after a missed anastomotic leak is high and is directly related to a delay in diagnosis; consider this diagnosis in a post-op bariatric patient even if they had an uneventful hospital and postoperative course. While most leaks happen early (within 30 days), delayed leaks are possible at any point after surgery. CT imaging and early consultation, particularly with a surgeon familiar with bariatric patients, are the key to diagnosis and successful management.

Marginal ulcer

Marginal ulcers typically form on the small bowel side of a gastrojejunostomy. Owing to the large number of asymptomatic patients, the true incidence of marginal ulcers is difficult to estimate with studies ranging from 1% to 16%.[67] Bariatric patients maintain a life-long risk for marginal ulcers with a mean time to onset of 12 months with most appearing by 2 years.

Although these ulcers may be asymptomatic initially, patients may eventually develop symptoms like dyspepsia, epigastric pain, and unexplained anemia. Fewer than 1% of marginal ulcers lead to perforation.[69] When this happens, however, they can manifest symptoms of perforation up to and including sepsis.

When a patient with a history of bariatric surgery presents with new gastritis symptoms or anemia, the diagnosis of marginal ulcer should be considered. With onset of symptoms suggestive of perforation, CT scan, broad-spectrum antibiotics, and surgical consultation should be aggressively pursued.

Bowel obstruction

Bariatric surgeries that only involve the stomach, such as SG and gastric banding, can develop bowel obstructions from adhesions in a process similar to other surgical procedures. When anatomic rearrangements are performed as are done in an RY (or the uncommonly performed duodenal switch), obstructions can additionally develop via intussusception and internal hernia.

Intussusception

Intussusception is a telescoping of the bowel. The lead point for intussusception after RY surgery is usually the jejunojejunal anastomosis site (see **Fig. 2**), occurring in either the proximal or distal segment.[67] Intussusception develops in 0.6% of RY patients with the mean interval between the surgery and presentation of 4.8 years.[70]

Signs and symptoms of intussusception mimic those of a bowel obstruction. CT scan should be obtained in suspected cases. Along with air-fluid levels, the classic finding on CT is the target sign, concentric circles of telescoping bowel seen in cross-section to form a "target" (see **Fig. 5**). A normal CT, however, does not adequately rule out intussusception and surgical consultation should be obtained in suspected cases.

Internal hernia

Bowel obstruction due to an internal hernia is most common after RY gastric bypass but can happen after other bariatric procedures involving GI bypass. Most studies report a 1% to 5% incidence of internal hernias post-RY surgery; however, the incidence was reported to be as high as 12.8% in one 10 years + observational study.[71,72]

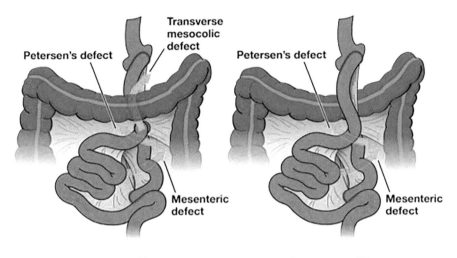

Retrocolic   **Antecolic**

Fig. 6. Possible sites of internal hernia after RY gastric bypass. (Alteiri et.al, American Society for Metabolic and Bariatric Surgery literature review on prevention, diagnosis, and management of internal hernias after Roux-en-Y gastric bypass, 2023, DOI:https://doi.org/10.1016/j.soard.2023.03.019.)

The internal hernia occurs as a result of the surgical defect created in the mesentery during the procedure (**Fig. 6**).

Patients with obstruction from an internal hernia are expected to have abdominal pain, which may be epigastric and/or radiate to the back. The symptoms are often intermittent, and the abdominal examination can appear benign unless the bowel has already become ischemic. To make the diagnosis more challenging, classic obstructive signs of nausea and vomiting may be absent, as the hernia may involve portions of the closed loop bypassed small bowel (**Fig. 7**).

A normal WBC count cannot rule out an internal hernia, with studies showing that leukocytosis was only present in 20% to 30% of patients with internal hernias. CT scans

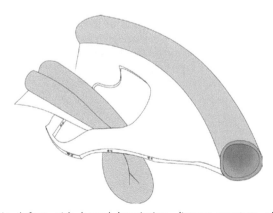

Fig. 7. Mesenteric defect with bowel herniation. (Image courtesy of Niels Olson via Wikicommons.)

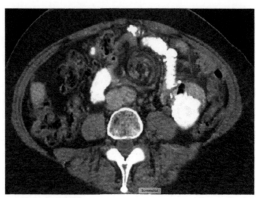

Fig. 8. Computed tomographic scans with IV contrast can reveal the classic "swirl" sign caused by twisting of the mesentery.

with intravenous (IV) contrast can reveal the classic "swirl" sign caused by twisting of the mesentery (**Fig. 8**); however, up to 30% of patients may have negative CT scans.[73] The addition of oral contrast (if tolerated) is not required to see the vascular swirl but may be useful in further delineating the associated bowel obstruction.

Because some cases of internal hernia present with intermittent symptoms, one can be lulled into a false sense of security. There are devastating consequences of missing strangulated bowel trapped in an internal hernia defect including bowel ischemia, perforation, and sepsis, with a mortality that can reach 50%.[74]

When a patient with a history of bariatric surgery (especially RY) presents with abdominal pain and intermittent signs of obstruction, imaging should be obtained along with consultation with general surgery. If your consultant is not familiar with bariatric surgical complications, you should seek consultation with the surgeon who did the procedure or discuss the case with another bariatric surgeon. Have a low threshold to transfer these patients if adequate surgical consultation is not available in a timely manner.

Adjustable gastric band
Although the AGB procedure is rarely performed today, it was a very popular procedure, and patients can still present with complications from a long-existing surgery. When slippage of the band occurs, a portion of the stomach can prolapse above the band causing an outlet obstruction and ischemia of the prolapsed segment. This complication carries a 22% lifetime risk of occurrence.[67]

While a plain radiograph can often diagnose a slipped AGB, a fluoroscopic swallow study is generally better. A CT scan is also helpful in the diagnosis.

CANCER
A new diagnosis of cancer is frequently made in the emergency department; persistent or recurrent abdominal or pelvic pain, weight loss, ongoing nausea, and vomiting or blood in the stool should prompt consideration abdominal imaging. Owing to metastasis, compression of adjacent structures, compromise of blood flow, and bony or central nervous system (CNS) invasion, almost any existing cancer can manifest with abdominal symptoms. For this article, we will focus on a specific cancer-related emergency that present with abdominal pain.

Typhlitis, or neutropenic enterocolitis, is a life-threatening condition that develops mostly, but not exclusively, in patients with hematologic malignancies who develop neutropenia and suppressed host defenses as a result of chemotherapy. The syndrome, which usually develops 2 to 3 weeks after chemotherapy, is characterized by fever, neutropenia (absolute neutrophil count <500 cells/microliter), and abdominal pain.[75] The pain may be anywhere in the abdomen but is more often in the right lower quadrant, involving the cecum (typhlon—Greek for cecum). The true incidence is not known, but it is estimated to affect around 5% of hospitalized patients with hematologic or solid tumors.[76] Additional symptoms can include diarrhea, bloating/distention, cramping, and bleeding. CT scanning is key in the diagnosis with bowel wall thickening greater than 4 mm for at least 30 cm of bowel length being a defining finding (**Fig. 9**).

The cause of typhlitis is multifactorial and includes impaired host defenses against mucosal invasion by intestinal bacteria along with pro-inflammatory cytokines and the effects of cytotoxic chemotherapy (**Table 2**).

Treatment by the EP begins with recognizing the diagnosis, followed by aggressive supportive care and the initiation of broad-spectrum antibiotics active against *Pseudomonas aeruginosa*, *Escherichia coli*, other enteric gram-negative bacilli, and anaerobes. Piperacillin-tazobactam or cefepime plus metronidazole is reasonable empiric therapy. In most cases, surgery is avoided; however, surgical consultation should be considered in patients with peritonitis, persistent bleeding, or decompensation despite aggressive resuscitation.

Although recent improvements in survival have been noted, the mortality rate for typhlitis is approximately 50%.[76]

DISCHARGING THE PATIENT WITH ABDOMINAL PAIN

Discharging a patient from the emergency department without a definitive diagnosis is common and should not be fraught with consternation but should be undertaken with a few important principles in mind:

- An explanation of the decision-making process should be documented.
- Reevaluation should be performed and documented.
- Abnormal vital signs should be rechecked and addressed in the decision-making portion of the documentation.

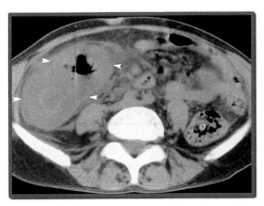

Fig. 9. CT scan demonstrating severe bowel wall thickening (*arrows*) greater than 4 mm for at least 30 cm of bowel length.

Table 2	
Criteria for diagnosis for typhlitis	
Criteria	**Finding**
Major	Neutropenia (ANC < 500)
	Bowel wall thickening >4 mm on CT or ultrasound for at least 30 cm of bowel
	Fever
Minor	Abdominal pain
	Abdominal distention
	Abdominal cramping
	Diarrhea
	Lower GI bleeding

Adapted from Gorschlüter M, Mey U, Strehl J, et al. Neutropenic enterocolitis in adults: Systematic analysis of evidence quality. Eur J Haematol. 2005;75(1). https://doi.org/10.1111/j.1600-0609.2005.00442.x.

- The diagnoses of constipation, gastroenteritis, indigestion, gas pains, function abdominal pain, and colic should be used with caution or chosen only after careful consideration and explanatory documentation.
- Normal or negatives tests should be explained to the patient in terms of their ability to rule out the disease.
- In cases where the diagnosis is uncertain and advanced imaging is not planned, the clinician should engage in shared decision-making with the patient, discussing the harms and benefits of not doing imaging early and returning to the question on a follow-up visit if the patient's symptoms become worse.
  - *Example: I discussed the pain with the patient and he and I agreed that we were not going to do any additional testing at this time since the pain was mild and improved with acetaminophen and antacids.*
- Good follow-up instructions with specific follow-up intervals should be given to the patient, for example, return for recheck within the next 24 hours. Further, the expected follow-up should be realistic and achievable within the system where the clinician practices.

Documentation in the chart does not have to be cumbersome or overly complicated. It can be as simple as follows:

Given patient's vague complaints of abdominal pain in the absence of anorexia or vomiting, I considered appendicitis but thought it to be low on the differential diagnosis and I felt imaging was low yield at this time in the course of illness. A recheck of the abdomen showed only mild discomfort that improved with acetaminophen and the patient's heart rate improved from 130 to 105 after fluids. I discussed the harms and benefits of my treatment plan of not doing imaging at this time, and the patient understands and is comfortable with this course. I instructed them to come back for a reevaluation in 12 to 24 hours or to return sooner if the pain becomes worse or is not improving as expected. The patient verbalized understanding of these instructions.

CLINICS CARE POINTS

- Appendicitis, biliary pathology, and vascular etiologies are the most common sources of litigation for abdominal pain
- "Rule-out" tests unfortunately do not exist in high-risk abdominal pain, and the careful emergency provider must know when a normal imaging study is not enough.

- Causes above the diaphragm and within the retroperitoneum are critically important to consider.
- Aging, diabetic, and immunocompromised patients present atypically and have higher rates of misdiagnosis, with cholecystitis and mesenteric ischemia far more common with age.
- Bariatric surgery complications and oncologic emergencies are common sources of medicolegal risk.

DISCLOSURE

The authors have nothing to disclose.

REFERENCES

1. Robinson DR, Gebhart GF. Inside information: The unique features of visceral sensation. Mol Interv 2008;8(5). https://doi.org/10.1124/mi.8.5.9.
2. Ferguson B, Geralds J, Petrey J, et al. Malpractice in Emergency Medicine—A Review of Risk and Mitigation Practices for the Emergency Medicine Provider. J Emerg Med 2018;55(5). https://doi.org/10.1016/j.jemermed.2018.06.035.
3. Cope Z. The early diagnosis of the acute abdomen. First. Henry Frowde and Hodder & Stoughton; 1921.
4. Alam HB. Cope's Early Diagnosis of the Acute Abdomen, 22nd Edition revised by William Silen. Oxford University Press; USA, 2011;24(4). 524. doi:10.1002/ca.21158.
5. Moffett P, Moore G. The standard of care: Legal history and definitions: The bad and good news. West J Emerg Med 2011;12(1).
6. Hall v Hillburn., Presented at the Mississippi Supreme Court, 1985.
7. McCourt v Abernathy. Presented at the South Carolina Supreme Court: 1995.
8. Johnston V, St. Francis Medical Center, Inc. Presented at the Louisiana Second Circuit Court of Appeal: 2001.
9. Osterwalder I, Özkan M, Malinovska A, et al. Acute abdominal pain: Missed diagnoses, extra-abdominal conditions, and outcomes. J Clin Med 2020;9(4). https://doi.org/10.3390/jcm9040899.
10. Rud B, Vejborg TS, Rappeport ED, et al. Computed tomography for diagnosis of acute appendicitis in adults. Cochrane Database Syst Rev 2019;2019(11). https://doi.org/10.1002/14651858.CD009977.pub2.
11. Henes FO, Pickhardt PJ, Herzyk A, et al. CT angiography in the setting of suspected acute mesenteric ischemia: prevalence of ischemic and alternative diagnoses. Abdominal Radiology 2017;42(4). https://doi.org/10.1007/s00261-016-0988-0.
12. Hlibczuk V, Dattaro JA, Jin Z, et al. Diagnostic accuracy of noncontrast computed tomography for appendicitis in adults: a systematic review. Ann Emerg Med 2010;55(1). https://doi.org/10.1016/j.annemergmed.2009.06.509.
13. Lourenco P, Brown J, Leipsic J, et al. The current utility of ultrasound in the diagnosis of acute appendicitis. Clin Imag 2016;40(5). https://doi.org/10.1016/j.clinimag.2016.03.012.
14. Pather V, Gosal P. A review of ultrasound for the diagnosis of acute appendicitis in adults. J Med Inform Decis Mak 2023;1(4). https://doi.org/10.14302/issn.2641-5526.jmid-23-4450.
15. Cho SU, Oh SK. Accuracy of ultrasound for the diagnosis of acute appendicitis in the emergency department: A systematic review. Medicine 2023;102(13). https://doi.org/10.1097/MD.0000000000033397.

16. Arruzza E, Milanese S, Li LSK, et al. Diagnostic accuracy of computed tomography and ultrasound for the diagnosis of acute appendicitis: A systematic review and meta-analysis. Radiography 2022;28(4). https://doi.org/10.1016/j.radi.2022.08.012.

17. Wertz JR, Lopez JM, Olson D, et al. Comparing the diagnostic accuracy of ultrasound and CT in evaluating acute cholecystitis. Am J Roentgenol 2018;211(2). https://doi.org/10.2214/AJR.17.18884.

18. Kiewiet JJS, Leeuwenburgh MMN, Bipat S, et al. A systematic review and meta-analysis of diagnostic performance of imaging in acute cholecystitis. Radiology 2012;264(3). https://doi.org/10.1148/radiol.12111561.

19. Bennett GL. Evaluating patients with right upper quadrant pain. Radiol Clin North Am 2015;53(6). https://doi.org/10.1016/j.rcl.2015.06.002.

20. Blachar A, Barnes S, Adam SZ, et al. Radiologists' performance in the diagnosis of acute intestinal ischemia, using MDCT and specific CT findings, using a variety of CT protocols. Emerg Radiol 2011;18(5). https://doi.org/10.1007/s10140-011-0965-4.

21. Aburahma AF, Stone PA, Srivastava M, et al. Mesenteric/celiac duplex ultrasound interpretation criteria revisited. J Vasc Surg 2012;55(2). https://doi.org/10.1016/j.jvs.2011.08.052.

22. Wattar B, Rimmer M, Rogozinska E, et al. Accuracy of imaging modalities for adnexal torsion: a systematic review and meta-analysis. BJOG 2021;128(1). https://doi.org/10.1111/1471-0528.16371.

23. Boendermaker AE, Coolsma CW, Emous M, et al. Efficacy of scheduled return visits for emergency department patients with non-specific abdominal pain. Emerg Med J 2018;35(8). https://doi.org/10.1136/emermed-2017-207338.

24. Mahajan P, Basu T, Pai CW, et al. Factors associated with potentially missed diagnosis of appendicitis in the emergency department. JAMA Netw Open 2020;3(3). https://doi.org/10.1001/jamanetworkopen.2020.0612.

25. Meltzer AC, Baumann BM, Chen EH, et al. Poor sensitivity of a modified alvarado score in adults with suspected appendicitis. Ann Emerg Med 2013;62(2). https://doi.org/10.1016/j.annemergmed.2013.01.021.

26. Diercks DB, Adkins EJ, Harrison N, et al. Clinical policy: critical issues in the evaluation and management of emergency department patients with suspected appendicitis: approved by ACEP Board of Directors February 1, 2023. Ann Emerg Med 2023;81(6). https://doi.org/10.1016/j.annemergmed.2023.01.015.

27. Karcz A, Holbrook J, Auerbach BS, et al. Preventability of malpractice claims in emergency medicine: A closed claims study. Ann Emerg Med 1990;19(8). https://doi.org/10.1016/S0196-0644(05)81559-8.

28. Gallaher JR, Charles A. A review of acute cholecystitis - reply. JAMA 2022;328(1). https://doi.org/10.1001/jama.2022.7771.

29. Fagenholz PJ, Fuentes E, Kaafarani H, et al. Computed tomography is more sensitive than ultrasound for the diagnosis of acute cholecystitis. Surg Infect 2015;16(5). https://doi.org/10.1089/sur.2015.102.

30. Cudnik MT, Darbha S, Jones J, et al. The diagnosis of acute mesenteric ischemia: A systematic review and meta-analysis. Acad Emerg Med 2013;20(11). https://doi.org/10.1111/acem.12254.

31. Gnanapandithan K, Feuerstadt P. Review article: mesenteric ischemia. Curr Gastroenterol Rep 2020;22(4). https://doi.org/10.1007/s11894-020-0754-x.

32. LeResche L. Defining gender disparities in pain management. Clin Orthop Relat Res 2011;469(7). https://doi.org/10.1007/s11999-010-1759-9.

33. Chen EH, Shofer FS, Dean AJ, et al. Gender disparity in analgesic treatment of emergency department patients with acute abdominal pain. Acad Emerg Med 2008;15(5). https://doi.org/10.1111/j.1553-2712.2008.00100.x.

34. Roth GA, Fleszar LG, Bryant AS, et al. Trends in State-Level Maternal Mortality by Racial and Ethnic Group in the United States. JAMA 2023;330(1). https://doi.org/10.1001/jama.2023.9043.

35. Joseph KS, Lisonkova S, Boutin A, et al. Maternal mortality in the United States: are the high and rising rates due to changes in obstetrical factors, maternal medical conditions, or maternal mortality surveillance? Am J Obstet Gynecol 2024. https://doi.org/10.1016/j.ajog.2023.12.038.

36. Crochet JR, Bastian LA, Chireau MV. Does this woman have an ectopic pregnancy? The rational clinical examination systematic review. JAMA 2013; 309(16). https://doi.org/10.1001/jama.2013.3914.

37. Mullany K, Minneci M, Monjazeb R, et al. Overview of ectopic pregnancy diagnosis, management, and innovation. Wom Health 2023;19. https://doi.org/10.1177/17455057231160349.

38. Hendriks E, Rosenberg R, Prine L. Ectopic pregnancy: diagnosis and management. Am Fam Physician 2020;101(10):599–606.

39. Houry D, Abbott JT. Ovarian torsion: a fifteen-year review. Ann Emerg Med 2001; 38(2). https://doi.org/10.1067/mem.2001.114303.

40. Tsafrir Z, Azem F, Hasson J, et al. Risk factors, symptoms, and treatment of ovarian torsion in children: the twelve-year experience of one center. J Minim Invasive Gynecol 2012;19(1). https://doi.org/10.1016/j.jmig.2011.08.722.

41. Huang C, Hong MK, Ding DC. A review of ovary torsion. Tzu Chi Med J 2017; 29(3). https://doi.org/10.4103/tcmj.tcmj_55_17.

42. Yen CF, Lin SL, Murk W, et al. Risk analysis of torsion and malignancy for adnexal masses during pregnancy. Fertil Steril 2009;91(5). https://doi.org/10.1016/j.fertnstert.2008.02.014.

43. Anders JF, Powell EC. Urgency of evaluation and outcome of acute ovarian torsion in pediatric patients. Arch Pediatr Adolesc Med 2005;159(6). https://doi.org/10.1001/archpedi.159.6.532.

44. Bardin R, Perl N, Mashiach R, et al. Prediction of adnexal torsion by ultrasound in women with acute abdominal pain. Ultraschall der Med 2020;41(6). https://doi.org/10.1055/a-1014-2593.

45. Workowski KA, Bachmann LH, Chan PA, et al. Sexually transmitted infections treatment guidelines, 2021. MMWR Recomm Rep (Morb Mortal Wkly Rep) 2021;70(4). https://doi.org/10.15585/mmwr.rr7004a1.

46. Williamson DA, Chen MY. Emerging and reemerging sexually transmitted infections. N Engl J Med 2020;382(21). https://doi.org/10.1056/nejmra1907194.

47. Han Y, Gong Y. Pulmonary embolism with abdominal pain as the chief complaint: A case report and literature review. Medicine 2019;98(44). https://doi.org/10.1097/MD.0000000000017791.

48. Hayes R. Abdominal pain: general imaging strategies. Eur Radiol Suppl 2004;14. https://doi.org/10.1007/s00330-003-2078-2.

49. Kasotakis G. Retroperitoneal and rectus sheath hematomas. Surg Clin 2014; 94(1). https://doi.org/10.1016/j.suc.2013.10.007.

50. Kwok CS, Kontopantelis E, Kinnaird T, et al. Retroperitoneal hemorrhage after percutaneous coronary intervention. Circ Cardiovasc Interv 2018;11(2). https://doi.org/10.1161/CIRCINTERVENTIONS.117.005866.

51. Caleo O, Bocchini G, Paoletta S, et al. Spontaneous non-aortic retroperitoneal hemorrhage: etiology, imaging characterization and impact of MDCT on

management. A multicentric study. Radiol Med 2015;120(1). https://doi.org/10.1007/s11547-014-0482-0.

52. Richards JR, McGahan JP. Focused assessment with sonography in trauma (FAST) in 2017: What radiologists can learn. Radiology 2017;283(1). https://doi.org/10.1148/radiol.2017160107.

53. Choinski K, Sanon O, Tadros R, et al. Review of malpractice lawsuits in the diagnosis and management of aortic aneurysms and aortic dissections. Vasc Endovasc Surg 2022;56(1). https://doi.org/10.1177/15385744211026455.

54. Hagan PG, Nienaber CA, Isselbacher EM, et al. The International Registry of Acute Aortic Dissection (IRAD): New insights into an old disease. J Am Med Assoc 2000;283(7). https://doi.org/10.1001/jama.283.7.897.

55. Tayal VS, Graf CD, Gibbs MA. Prospective study of accuracy and outcome of emergency ultrasound for abdominal aortic aneurysm over two years. Acad Emerg Med 2003;10(8). https://doi.org/10.1197/aemj.10.8.867.

56. Reed K, MD F, Curtis L, et al. Aortic emergencies - Part II: abdominal aneurysms and aortic trauma. Emerg Med Pract 2006;8(3).

57. Azhar B, Patel SR, Holt PJE, et al. Misdiagnosis of ruptured abdominal aortic aneurysm: systematic review and meta-analysis. J Endovasc Ther 2014;21(4). https://doi.org/10.1583/13-4626MR.1.

58. Marien T, Miller NL. Treatment of the infected stone. Urol Clin 2015;42(4). https://doi.org/10.1016/j.ucl.2015.05.009.

59. Gaither TW, Copp HL. State appellant cases for testicular torsion: case review from 1985 to 2015. J Pediatr Urol 2016;12(5). https://doi.org/10.1016/j.jpurol.2016.03.008.

60. Vasconcelos-Castro S, Soares-Oliveira M. Abdominal pain in teenagers: beware of testicular torsion. J Pediatr Surg 2020;55(9). https://doi.org/10.1016/j.jpedsurg.2019.08.014.

61. Baker LA, Sigman D, Mathews RI, et al. An analysis of clinical outcomes using color Doppler testicular ultrasound for testicular torsion. Pediatrics 2000;105(3). https://doi.org/10.1542/peds.105.3.604.

62. Ota K, Fukui K, Oba K, et al. The role of ultrasound imaging in adult patients with testicular torsion: a systematic review and meta-analysis. J Med Ultrason 2019;46(3). https://doi.org/10.1007/s10396-019-00937-3.

63. Vasdev N, Chadwick D, Thomas D. The acute pediatric scrotum: presentation, differential diagnosis and management. Curr Urol 2012;6(2). https://doi.org/10.1159/000343509.

64. Laurell H, Hansson LE, Gunnarsson U. Acute abdominal pain among elderly patients. Gerontology 2006;52(6). https://doi.org/10.1159/000094982.

65. Kanbakan A, Cakmak F, Ipekci A, et al. Geriatric mortality risk factors in emergency department for non-traumatic abdominal pain. Bratislava Med J 2023;124(9). https://doi.org/10.4149/BLL_2023_109.

66. ASMBS. Estimate of bariatric surgery numbers, 2011-2019 | American society for metabolic and bariatric surgery. Asmbs. Available at: https://asmbs.org/resources/estimate-of-bariatric-surgery-numbers/. Accessed 2023.

67. Altieri MS, Rogers A, Afaneh C, et al. Bariatric emergencies for the general surgeon. Surg Obes Relat Dis 2023;19(5). https://doi.org/10.1016/j.soard.2023.02.007.

68. Choudhry AJ, Haddad NN, Martin M, et al. Medical malpractice in bariatric surgery: a review of 140 medicolegal claims. J Gastrointest Surg 2017;21(1). https://doi.org/10.1007/s11605-016-3273-1.

69. Carr WRJ, Mahawar KK, Balupuri S, et al. An evidence-based algorithm for the management of marginal ulcers following Roux-en-Y gastric bypass. Obes Surg 2014;24(9). https://doi.org/10.1007/s11695-014-1293-z.

70. Papasavas P, Docimo S, Oviedo RJ, et al. Biliopancreatic access following anatomy-altering bariatric surgery: a literature review. Surg Obes Relat Dis 2022;18(1). https://doi.org/10.1016/j.soard.2021.09.011.

71. Obeid NR, Malick W, Concors SJ, et al. Long-term outcomes after Roux-en-Y gastric bypass: 10- to 13-year data. Surg Obes Relat Dis 2016;12(1). https://doi.org/10.1016/j.soard.2015.04.011.

72. Al Harakeh AB, Kallies KJ, Borgert AJ, et al. Bowel obstruction rates in antecolic/antegastric versus retrocolic/retrogastric Roux limb gastric bypass: A meta-analysis. Surg Obes Relat Dis 2016;12(1). https://doi.org/10.1016/j.soard.2015.02.004.

73. Comeau E, Gagner M, Inabnet WB, et al. Symptomatic internal hernias after laparoscopic bariatric surgery. Surg Endosc 2005;19(1). https://doi.org/10.1007/s00464-003-8515-0.

74. Lanzetta MM, Masserelli A, Addeo G, et al. Internal hernias: a difficult diagnostic challenge. Review of CT signs and clinical findings. Acta Biomed 2019;90. https://doi.org/10.23750/abm.v90i5-S.8344.

75. Snydman DR, Nesher L, Rolston KVI. Neutropenic enterocolitis, a growing concern in the era of widespread use of aggressive chemotherapy. Clin Infect Dis 2013;56(5). https://doi.org/10.1093/cid/cis998.

76. Gorschlüter M, Mey U, Strehl J, et al. Neutropenic enterocolitis in adults: systematic analysis of evidence quality. Eur J Haematol 2005;75(1). https://doi.org/10.1111/j.1600-0609.2005.00442.x.

Legal Risk to the Emergency Medicine Resident in Training and Attending Supervisors

Nicole Tyczynska, MD[a],*, Rebecca E. Younker, Esq, PA-C[b,1]

KEYWORDS

- Resident physician • Supervision • Medical malpractice • Litigation risk • Telehealth

KEY POINTS

- Medical malpractice in the United States is a significant issue that influences the practice patterns of residents and supervising attendings, leaving unanswered questions about the best balance between graded resident autonomy and supervision.
- Determining the actual legal risk for residents in training and their supervising physicians is difficult due to numerous variables that make collecting comprehensive data on medical malpractice claims near impossible.
- The use of telemedicine has substantially increased, posing unique challenges to residents and supervising attendings who are learning to interact with this novel modality of delivering health care.
- Residents and supervising attendings can minimize litigation risk by ensuring good bedside manners, staying updated on new medical developments, having strong open communication, and confirming proper documentation on patient charts.

INTRODUCTION

Medical malpractice is a prevalent issue in the United States, with an estimated 20,000 medical malpractice lawsuits filed annually. In 2022, 31% of practicing US physicians reported being involved in at least one malpractice case in their career, with emergency physicians coming in above the national average at 46.8%.[1] Medical liability costs the US health care system an estimated US$55.6 billion a year, averaging 2.4% of total annual health care spending in 2010.[2] Medical malpractice expenses go beyond the individual physicians they impact, having far-reaching ramifications

[a] University of Pennsylvania at Pennsylvania Hospital and Penn Presbyterian Medical Center;
[b] Troutman Pepper
[1] Sq 18th and Two Logan Square, 3000 Arch Street, Philadelphia, PA 19103, USA
* Corresponding author: 800 Spruce Street, Philadelphia, PA 19107.
E-mail address: Nicoletyczy@gmail.com

Emerg Med Clin N Am 43 (2025) 115–130
https://doi.org/10.1016/j.emc.2024.05.020
emed.theclinics.com

on society. Beyond the monetary cost, fear over the risks of practicing medicine as a trainee influences the minds of young physicians, priming them to adopt defensive medicine strategies in a formative time in their careers when they are developing their risk tolerance level and solidifying future practice patterns.[3] Fear of litigation can also cause the supervising attending to curtail trainees' independent practice and restrict access to performing challenging procedures, thwarting skills development. The lack of formalized medical school and residency curriculum on the medical-legal system, including understanding malpractice risk and employment of legal risk mitigation strategies, can amplify these practices.

This review describes the legal risk to the residents in training and the supervising attending physician. This review also reviews the legal risks associated with practicing and precepting residents via telemedicine.

LEGAL NOMENCLATURE AND STUDY LIMITATIONS
Nomenclature

Since most physicians do not have a double major in law (kudos to those of you who do), understanding legal literature can be difficult for those unfamiliar with the nomenclature. It is important to grasp certain fundamental principles to understand key information and conclusions from the studies described in this review. A legal case begins as a "claim" against a physician. This claim can be mediated before reaching the court system. This is called arbitration. Most times, this occurs in a pre-court setting, either through a hospital's internal legal mediation system or as a negotiation between 2 groups of lawyers. The goal is to negotiate a settlement before a case goes to court. Most cases do not go to court. If arbitration results in a payment to the patient, this is called a "paid claim." Only paid claims are legally required to be logged in the National Provider Database (NPDB). Claims that are not paid out to the patient are not reliably trackable, therefore, limiting our ability to analyze all reasons for medical malpractice claims. Civil law that includes medical malpractice law is termed "Tort law." Tort reform is the term used to describe changes in laws that affect the medical malpractice climate within your state.

Study Limitations

Literature on risks associated with practicing medicine as a trainee (student, resident, or fellow), as well as literature on risks associated with being a supervising physician working with a trainee, is heterogeneous. Multiple studies exist; however, no 2 studies compare the same cohort of study participants, making it difficult to collate data and make conclusions. Further, these studies pull data from various sources. Legal databases, like Westlaw and Lexis, are incomplete due to court and jurisdiction limitations; the NPDB only provides documents for paid claims; insurance claims data, although it does look at both paid and unpaid claims, is susceptible to coding bias.

Table 1 presents the core group of studies reviewed for this article and describes the data sources used, the characteristics of the populations studied, and the key conclusions.

LEGAL RISK TO THE EMERGENCY MEDICINE RESIDENT IN TRAINING
Emergency Medicine Resident: Legal Epidemiology

There were 9346 emergency medicine (EM) residents in 2022 to 2023, making up 6% of the 158,079 total active residents in the United States.[4]

It is not common for an EM resident to be named in a malpractice case that results in payment (72% of claims do not result in indemnity)[2] or that reaches the public court

Table 1
Core group of studies reviewed and data sources used, the characteristics of the populations studied, and the key conclusions for this study

Article/Year	Data Source	Population Studied	Key Data Identified and Conclusions
Poyorena 2023 Review of medical malpractice involving EM Trainees	Westlaw Database 1982–2017 Only shows subset of federal and state cases that were tried in court	EM trainees Medical student to fourth year resident	• 60 cases (trial cases) • Errors (diagnostic 61%, treatment 21%, procedures 16%) • 35% of cases—no attending involvement • Very low likelihood of a claim going to trial
Antkowiak 2023 Malpractice cases involving EM Trainees, APPs, and Attendings	Candello Database 2010–2019 Paid + unpaid claims Only captured about one-third of cases in the United States	EM providers APPs vs trainee vs EM attending "Physician extender" is defined as an APP or trainee helping the attending	• 5854 cases over 10 y • 78% claims had no "physician extender" • 9.1% claims involved a trainee • Cases with trainees highest gross indemnity • APPs + trainees: 21% of malpractice cases, 33% of total gross indemnity paid
Glover 2020 Characteristics of paid claims among Residents in USA from 2001-2015	NPDB 2001–2015 Paid malpractice claims. This database captures 100% of paid claims	All specialties Trainees All interns vs residents vs fellows	• Overall risk for trainees is low 0.76/1000 resident years • Paid claims rates fell 52% from 2001 to 2015 • Trainee paid claims rates were lower than attending rates
Myers 2020 Examination of medical malpractice claims involving physician trainees from 2012-2016	CRICO Comparative Benchmark System (CBS) Looked at "closed" claims from 2012–2016 All claims—paid and unpaid	Trainees—all specialties Compare characteristics of claims where trainees were directly involved in patient harm events vs controls	• 81% named resident (vs student or fellow) • Trainee more likely to be named if directly involved in harm event (32% vs 9% control) • Care in ED increased risk • 24% lack of supervision

(continued on next page)

Table 1
(continued)

Article/Year	Data Source	Population Studied	Key Data Identified and Conclusions
Myers 2020 Characteristic of medical malpractice claims involving EM physicians	CRICO CBS 2007–2016 All claims—paid and unpaid	Attending providers All specialties (not trainees) EM physician subset analyzed	• 74% procedural • 5% claims = ED docs • Diagnosis-related allegations –58% • 31% EM claims are paid • Payment more likely for procedure-related
Gurley 2018 Comparison of EM Malpractice cases involving residents to non-residents	CRICO Comparative Benchmarking System 2009–2013 Open and closed EM cases	Trainee vs not trainee EM cases naming a resident vs cases *not* naming a resident	• 87% nonresident • 13% residents named • Resident cases incurred lower payments on average, but 66% of resident cases vs 57% involved high-severity claims
Jena 2011 Malpractice Risk according to specialty	Malpractice data from large professional liability insurer	All physicians—25 specialties *Not trainees*	Top 3 contributing factors: • Clinical judgment • Communication • Documentation • Each year, 7.4% of all doctors have malpractice claim • 78% of claims are not paid • By age 65 y, 75% of physicians in low-risk specialties had claims • 99% of physicians in high-risk specialties had claims

system (94% of cases settle, 3.5% go to court, and 2.5% have unknown outcomes).[5] Although residents are named in malpractice cases, it is more common for plaintiffs to target the supervising attending or the hospital that employs the resident.[6]

In a study reviewing all medical malpractice court cases involving trainees in the emergency department (ED), Poyorena and colleagues found only 60 cases reported in the Westlaw legal database between 1982 and 2017. This study, although published recently, reports on older data but simultaneously highlights that, over 35 years, only 60 trainee-related cases made it as far as court. Of these cases involving EM trainees that were tried in court, 30% of juries decided in favor of the patient, 42% in favor of the physician, and 28% of cases settled.[7]

Another large analysis of all paid claims registered in the NPDB between 2001 and 2015 showed only 75 EM-based paid claims recorded at that time, with a malpractice claim rate of 1.03 claims for every 1000 resident years (95% confidence interval [CI]: 0.81, 1.29).[5]

Despite evidence gleaned from these few studies, it is nearly impossible to accurately quantify how many residents are sued every year or what percentages of those residents "lose" as there is no one absolute database that logs all malpractice claims filed against residents or attendings. Data sources that collect information regarding medical malpractice cases are imperfect; for example, Westlaw and Lexis, which are legal repositories of select cases tried in front of a judge and jury, only account for federal and about 50% of state court cases. Moreover, these databases are comprised of court cases selected by court reporters to be published and do not require the published cases to contain standardized amounts of information about each case. They are written for a lay audience and often do not contain complete accounts of medical information, making data analysis difficult. In addition, most malpractice claims never make it to court as health care systems have elaborate internal networks for claims mediation and arbitration to settle claims within an "internal court system," thereby excluding them from being registered in these databases. Even the NPDB, a federal government-run database of claims paid for licensed health care practitioners, only mandates that claims resulting in payments be registered. It does not account for medical malpractice claims that do not result in payment or that are paid on an institution's behalf, effectively "shielding" individual practitioners and making the data incomplete.

Some large retrospective reviews have relied on queries of medical malpractice claims databases created by companies such as the Controlled Risk Insurance Company (CRICO), which captures both paid and unpaid claims. However, data from these reviews are limited because they rely on insurance claim data collected by medical coders extracting data from International Classification of Diseases 10th (ICD-10) revision codes. This method makes data collection susceptible to coding error and bias.

In short, there is no way to account for all the residents named but dropped from cases or involved in cases that did not result in an indemnity payment to the plaintiff.[8]

Comparison of Risk: Legal Liability for Emergency Medicine Residents versus Other Specialties

A study by Glover and colleagues, which analyzed paid malpractice claims across all specialties for both residents and attendings from 2001 to 2015, showed that 1248 paid claims were submitted to the NPDB on behalf of 1194 residents, with a majority (95.7%) of residents having only one claim. The rate of resident malpractice claims is 0.76 claims per 1000 resident-years. The highest risk resident specialties were obstetrics and gynecology (2.96) and neurosurgery (2.01), while the lowest risk were pathology (0.12) and psychiatry/neurology (0.15), followed by pediatrics (0.22). EM ranked

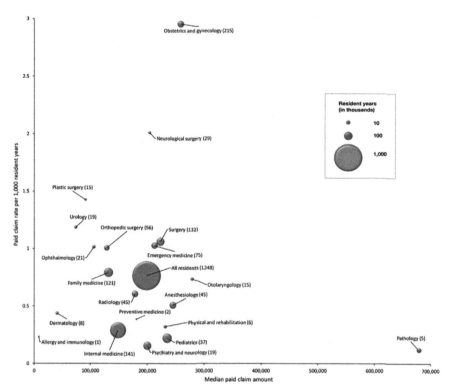

Fig. 1. Paid malpractice claim rates on behalf of resident physicians, median payment amounts, and total resident year risk, by specialty, in the United States, 2001 to 2015. Payment amounts are inflation adjusted to US$2015. Numbers in parentheses are the total number of paid claims in that specialty. (*From* Glover M, McGee GW, Wilkinson DS, et al. Characteristics of Paid Malpractice Claims among Resident Physicians from 2001 to 2015 in the United States. Academic Medicine. 2020;95(2):255–262. https://doi.org/10.1097/ACM. 0000000000003039; with permission.)

higher than the overall average but still well below the top at-risk specialties, with a rate of 1.03 claims for every 1000 resident years (95% CI: 0.81, 1.29) (**Fig. 1**).[5]

Resident Malpractice Payment Trends

Malpractice claims have decreased over time. In the same study by Glover and colleagues, there was an overall decreased claims rate of 52% when comparing the time period of 2011 - 2015 to 2001 - 2005 with a statistically significant reduction in the rate of claims paid in EM-based cases from 2001 to 2015.[5]

The median inflation-adjusted malpractice payment amount for resident cases during this time was US$199,014 and did not significantly change over the 15 year study period. Similarly, the proportion of catastrophic claims (11.1%), defined as claims paying more than US$1 million, and the percentage of small claims (33.1%), defined as less than US$100,000, stayed consistent.[5]

Causes of Medical Malpractice Claims that Name Residents

The most common reasons for which EM residents were named in malpractice cases involved diagnostic (62%), treatment (21%), and procedural errors (16%). The top clinical categories of malpractice were neurologic (22%), infectious (22%), traumatic

(18%), and cardiac (17%) in one study.[7] In another study, procedure-related complications were noted in 32% of resident malpractice cases, with vascular and spinal procedures being most common.[9]

In a study of claims closed between 2012 and 2016 involving trainees of all subspecialties, residents were much more likely to be named as a defendant in the case (32%) if they were directly involved in the patient harm event than if they were not directly involved in the harm event (9%). Inadequate supervision contributed to 24% of these cases in which a trainee was directly involved in harm to a patient, and most of these claims were procedure-related (74%). The most common error was puncture or laceration during a procedure. A multivariable regression analysis from this same dataset showed that trainees were most likely to be involved in harmful events when performing procedures (and when delivering care in the ED).[10]

Issues with clinical judgment, communication, and documentation were differentiated as important contributing causes of malpractice risk.[9] Claims resulting in medical error were more likely to involve "excessive workloads, handoff issues, technical competence, and lack of supervision."[11]

Lack of attending supervision was a large contributor in a study of cases tried in court, with 35% alleging no attending involvement before the malpractice event and unclear or minimal attending involvement in 47% of cases.[7]

Standard of Care: Resident versus Attending Physician

Standard of care is the cornerstone of how physicians are tried and whether they are found guilty of malpractice within their level of training and field.

For a patient to have a legitimate medical malpractice claim against a resident or supervising attending, the patient must prove the following:

1. The patient has a recognizable injury.
2. There is a duty of care (ie, legitimate patient–provider relationship).
3. There is a breach of this duty of care (ie, deviation from the "standard of care").
4. The breach of care is the proximate causation of the injury.

Standard of care is defined as "a measure by which a health care provider's professional conduct is evaluated in the legal system." The definition as to how the law should view a resident has been debated for years. Since 1957, when the standard of care was defined as that of an "intern," the perceived competency of a resident has evolved from being that of a "physician of ordinary skill, care and diligence" such as an attending general practitioner, to what is currently considered the standard of care, which is that residents are viewed as practicing to the same standard as an attending specialist in their field. Resident liability extends to the attending specialist supervising the resident and the hospital, which has a legal duty to provide supervised care to the patient. Since attendings are directly responsible and serve as quality control, in theory, outcomes should not hinge on the level of resident training but rather be held to the standard of the highest provider.[6]

As a result, currently, in most states, a resident physician is held to the same standard of care as an attending physician in the same specialty.

Minimizing Resident Litigation Risk

Above all, residents should be aware that there is no guaranteed way to avoid a lawsuit and that, in some instances, a patient may initiate legal action regardless of the quality of care or the health care provider involved.[12]

However, there are proactive measures that can be taken to decrease the probability of being named.

1. Good bedside manner: High-quality bedside manner has consistently been mentioned within the medicolegal community as a strategy to avoid litigation. The foundation of good bedside manner is effective communication, which may even be considered one and the same. It is important not only for improved patient satisfaction but in the case of an adverse outcome, it may also decrease the risk of legal action being initiated. Beyond the universal sentiment, good bedside manner preventing litigation has been frequently studied.[12–14]

2. Stay updated on new medical developments to adhere to the proper care standard: While adhering to the proper standard of care and practice guidelines may not prevent an initial lawsuit, maintaining such adherence can significantly reduce the chances of a successful lawsuit.

3. Understand hospital policies and resident support programs: Residents should understand what support their hospital and residency programs offer. Academic centers are designed to foster an environment that takes action to prevent litigation. Residents can ask questions such as
   - What support systems do the hospitals have to cope with errors and malpractice claims?
   - Does the hospital have any verbiage during the patient registration process that specifies that patients will be cared for by physicians in training?

4. Documentation: Proper documentation allows for good communication among providers as well as adherence to regulatory and insurance requirements. Proper documentation is the main evidence utilized in litigation to show what was done or not done. A popular saying is, "if you didn't document it, it didn't happen." Although not necessarily correct, residents should accurately document important and relevant aspects of the ED encounter. Particularly important, residents should document patient education, discharge instructions, and specific return precautions. There is a relatively new increase in cases involving informed consent as the basis for medical malpractice claims.[15,16] Many common ED procedures require written consent; residents should learn the hospitals' policies for procedures to ensure they are following the proper informed consent protocol.

5. Be the "squeaky wheel": Residents should be vocal when they feel they are practicing outside their comfort level. In many lawsuits involving residents, the basis for litigation is lack of adequate supervision.[7,10,17,18] In 2 studies of resident-centered litigation in EM, approximately one-fourth (24.7% Antkowiak, 30% Kachalia) of cases involved claims of inadequate supervision.[18,19] Although there is no high-quality evidence that supervision reduces mortality, it is associated with a significantly reduced risk of complication during nonsurgical invasive procedures.[20]

In 2008, the Institute of Medicine (IOM) increased supervision requirements for physicians in training and recommended limiting resident duty hours and improving wellness initiatives to decrease fatigue. They also mandated 24/7 in-house supervision for all critical care services, including EDs, and direct supervision was expected for all high-acuity cases.[21] This IOM report resulted in increased federal oversight of the Accreditation Council of Graduate Medical Education (ACGME) and eventually led to the infamous 2010 ACGME practice changes, including duty hour restrictions and enhanced supervision requirements for residency programs.[20]

LEGAL RISK TO THE SUPERVISING ATTENDING
General Medical Malpractice Risk for Attendings

Most US physicians will be named in a malpractice claim at some point in their career. By the age of 65 years, 75% of doctors practicing in "low-risk" specialties will be part of a malpractice claim, and up to 99% of physicians in "high-risk" specialties will be named. Contrary to popular belief, EM does not rank among the top high-risk physician specialties, coming in at just above the national average for legal risk for "all physicians." According to Jena and colleagues, EM physicians have a 7.5% annual risk of being involved in a malpractice claim.[22] Although frequency of claims against EM doctors has been increasing steadily over time, the United States has experienced an overall decrease in civil liability cases that end up in court in the 15 years from 2000 to 2015, with reports from the National Center for State Courts showing that tort lawsuits decreased 21% in that time.[23] As a provider, it is important that you understand that your likelihood of being named, and even more so the likelihood of the case being successful for the patient, relies heavily on your state's tort laws and limitations within and how litigious a region you practice in. One study found a paid claim rate of 5.5 per 1000 physicians among the bottom tertile of states compared to 14.6 per 1000 physicians for states in the top tertile.[24]

Supervising Attending Medical Malpractice Risks when Working with Residents

It seems instinctive to presume that working with a trainee increases the probability of malpractice for a supervisor. However, no studies directly answer whether working with a resident increases an attending's risk of being named in a legal case.

Overall, the risk of being involved in a malpractice claim that results in payment is extremely low for ED residents (1.03 paid claims/1000 resident-years) and statistically decreased from 2001 to 2015.[5] There have been a handful of large retrospective database reviews comparing characteristics of cases involving residents to ones where residents are not named.

In a study by Gurley in 2018, looking at 845 EM cases, only 13% of cases involved residents. Within this cohort of resident cases, the attending was also named 60% of the time. Resident cases, compared to attending-only cases, incurred lower payments on average (US$51,163 with resident named vs US$156,212 without resident named). However, a higher percentage of resident cases were associated with "high-severity outcomes" such as death or permanent disability (66% in resident-involved claims vs 57% in no-resident claims).

In a large case-control study from Myers and colleagues of 30,973 malpractice claims involving trainees from all physician specialties, only 581 were classified as cases that directly involved trainees in patient harm events. Eighty-one percent of the trainees were residents, 13% were fellows, and 6% were both residents and fellows. Trainees were much more likely to be named as the defendant in cases where they were directly related to the harm event (32%) than in cases where the trainees were not directly involved in the harm caused to the patient (9%).[10]

In a 2023 study by Antkowiak comparing malpractice cases involving EM attendings, residents, and advanced practice providers (APPs), only 9.1% of claims involved a resident versus 78% of claims that were made against attendings practicing with "no physician extender." In comparison to data by Gurley, this study noted that resident cases accounted for the highest-paid claims on average. Reasons for the higher gross indemnity associated with trainee cases could be due to the following:

- "Complications" were the most common final diagnosis.
- Issues with "technical skills" were more common in trainees.
- Higher percentage of systems-related contributors.[18]

Common Themes in Malpractice Cases Involving Trainees (Residents and Fellows)

- Singh and colleagues 2007 (Trainees of all subspecialties): Claims resulting in medical error were more likely to involve "excessive workloads, handoff issues, technical competence, and lack of supervision."[11]
- Gurley and colleagues 2018 (EM residents and attendings): "Failure or delay in diagnosis" followed by "medical treatment" were the most frequent allegations. Procedure-related complications were noted in 32% of resident malpractice cases, with vascular and spinal procedures being more commonly cited than in attending cases. Cardiac diagnoses were the most common "final diagnosis" in resident-related malpractice cases. Issues with clinical judgment, communication, and documentation were differentiated as important contributing causes of malpractice risk.[9]
- Myers 2020 (Trainees of all subspecialties): Inadequate supervision contributed to 24% of cases, 74% of which involved lack of supervision during a procedure. Trainees were most likely to be involved in harmful events when performing procedures (odds ratio [OR] = 1.58, 95% CI: 1.27, 1.96) or when delivering care in an emergency room (OR = 1.65, 95% CI: 1.43, 1.91).[10]
- Poyorena 2023 (EM trainees): Lack of attending supervision was a large contributor to these court cases, with 35% of cases alleging no attending involvement before malpractice event and unclear or minimal attending involvement in 47% of cases. Similar to other studies, failure to diagnose (62%), inappropriate treatment (22%), and procedural error (15%) were the top alleged errors.[7]
- Atkowiak 2023 (EM trainees): Trainees had a higher proportion of claims with "complications" listed as the diagnosis. Trainees had a higher percentage of allegations related to the following "contributing factors": clinical environment, technical skill, clinical systems, and documentation.[18]

Minimizing Supervising Attending Litigation Risk

1. Know where the risks in EM lie: Most EM-based claims are related to diagnostic errors, followed by treatment-related and procedural errors. The most common severity of outcomes was death, and residents are more likely to be associated with high-severity outcomes.[7,9,10,18] Catastrophic claims were statistically higher for residents (11.1%) than for attending physicians (8.0%, $P < .001$).[5] Highly reported areas of performance concerns included high-risk cardiovascular pathologies like acute myocardial infarction, pulmonary embolism, and cardiac arrest—the top 3 final diagnoses in EM malpractice claims—each accounting for 2% of claims (intubation as well as vascular and spinal procedures were other notable reported areas).[25] Knowing these areas are the highest contributors to claims will allow physicians to keep vigilant surrounding these risks.

2. Documentation for supervising attendings: Attendings should be familiar with their supervisory note template and ensure their level of supervision aligns with what is stated. Reimbursements, particularly from Medicare, depend on appropriate supervision.[26] If the insurance company will only pay an attending rate if XYZ is done, then it is likely that doing XYZ is enough supervision to mitigate legal risk. Further, attendings should thoroughly review what is written before adding the supervisory attestation to resident notes. Electronic medical record audits can see the time an attending spends reviewing each note, which could be used against them if not enough time is allotted to plausibly review a note.

3. Proper supervision: Treating residents with respect creates an open environment that decreases the risk of miscommunication between attendings and residents. Clinical supervision should provide trainees with monitoring, guidance, and feedback while

ensuring patient safety.[27] Past studies have shown that malpractice claims with explicit medical errors involving trainees were more likely to be affected by excessive workloads, handoff issues, lack of technical competence, and poor supervision.[11] It is important for attending physicians to afford their residents a graduated level of responsibility and supervision commensurate with their level of experience, as supported by the ACGME guidelines.[28] Attendings should also lead by example regarding self-care, fatigue mitigation, and work–life balance.

4. Good bedside manners expand to residents: Physicians who develop strong physician–patient trust relationships are less likely to be named in malpractice cases.[29] It is important to teach residents the value of honest reporting of errors in their practice, as apologies make patients more likely to forgive physician errors and less likely to pursue litigation.[30] Attendings can lessen their legal risk with residents by expanding good bedside manner practices to their residents.[31,32]

LEGAL RISK OF RESIDENTS PRACTICING TELEHEALTH

Telemedicine has been a resource since before the coronavirus disease 2019 (COVID-19) pandemic, but initial growth was thwarted by poor reimbursement structures for direct-to-consumer (DTC) tele-visits.[25] The pandemic fast-tracked telehealth as one of the Nation's top priorities.[31] An estimated 42% of the US population utilized telemedicine services during the pandemic, solidifying telehealth as an indispensable health care service.[33]

Telehealth-related Medical Malpractice Claims

Not much legal information is available about telehealth civil lawsuits. A research study by Kvedar in 2019 showed no malpractice cases were held against providers involved in DTC telemedicine. This lack of data may be due to the specific cohort of patients served via telehealth. DTC telemedicine encounters are typically lower acuity and lower risk. They are, therefore, less likely to end in litigation, or if a claim is made, it is more likely to be settled precourt through arbitration or mediation. Higher risk specialties, such as neurosurgery, are rarely available as a telehealth service, and other high-stakes encounters, such as telestroke consultations, are not provided directly to patients outside of a hospital setting. Many telehealth companies have risk-lowering practices such as bans on prescribing controlled substances and policies that redirect patients with concerning symptoms to seek in-person care.[34]

Standard of Care for Telemedicine Training and Practice

During the COVID-19 pandemic, the speed with which telehealth services expanded and the lack of clear practice guidelines left providers at all stages of their careers to implement telemedicine "ad hoc."[35]

Due to the public health emergency, pandemic-related laws were drafted to help protect clinicians, and Center for Medicare and Medicaid Services (CMS) regulations decreased supervisory requirements during that time. This gave organizations such as the American Medical Association ("AMA"), Association of American Medical Colleges ("AAMC"), and ACGME time to develop guidelines for telemedicine training as well as practice-based competencies.

These organizations agreed on a need to standardize telehealth education and training for the clinician workforce. The AAMC established a Telehealth Advisory Committee to identify skills needed to practice high-quality telemedicine by all physicians, irrespective of specialty. This same working group created 6 comprehensive telehealth competencies to define a standard of care for encounters and training of young providers.[36]

As most lawsuits extend from a breach of standard of care practices, it will be increasingly expected that residents understand their telehealth core competencies and whether they are practicing within their expected level of competency.

Supervision of Residents Practicing Telehealth

The AMA Council of Medical Education drafted an executive summary as early as 2016 outlining the importance of integrating telemedicine training into Undergraduate Medical Education (UME), Graduate Medical Education (GME), and Continuing Medical Education (CME) for all providers.[37]

Precepting in the realm of telemedicine has been coined "teleprecepting." It involves either remotely precepting a resident with a patient or providing in-person supervision to a resident taking care of a patient via telehealth.[38]

ACGME common program requirements support teleprecepting, stating that if a program can demonstrate that an "appropriate level of supervision is in place for all residents," it supports supervision via "telephonic and/or electronic modalities" both in real-time and as a "post-hoc review of resident-delivered care with feedback."[39]

There is no one set of national supervisory guidelines specific to telemedicine and available guidelines defer to supervision that would be "appropriate to the level of resident training." The ACGME's "Specialty-Specific Program Requirements: Direct Supervision Using Telecommunication Technology" document empowers specialty-specific review committees to further define expectations related to direct supervision.[40]

Telemedicine does not currently exist as a required rotation for EM although some institutions offer it as an elective and have developed center-specific supervisory rules as a result.

Since January 1, 2024, increased CMS regulations surrounding billing for supervising services have tightened restrictions on attending supervision of resident telehealth encounters. This may lead to changes in the intensity of supervision required for resident-performed encounters.[41]

Minimizing Litigation Risk Associated with Telemedicine Visits

- The legal risk of practicing or supervising telemedicine is currently no different than the legal risk of being a resident or attending in any other capacity.
- As a resident in training or an attending new to telehealth, the legal risk can be minimized by understanding the expected clinical competencies.
- Understand the inherent risks unique to telehealth and the laws surrounding telehealth practice.

The Center for Connected Health Policy ("CCHP") Web site is a repository of information on state-specific telehealth policy. The goal of CCHP is to "track and compile telehealth-related laws and regulations" and to make "telehealth policy more accessible to everyone."[42] The US Department of Health and Human Services (HHS) Web site on telehealth can also serve as a source of updates on best practice guidelines, licensure requirements, Healthcare Insurance Portability and Accountability Act (HIPAA) compliance, telehealth billing, and policy changes.[43] Be mindful that CMS and HHS may change certain regulations and that some telehealth flexibilities originally enacted during the pandemic are temporary.[44]

SUMMARY

Medical malpractice is an expected and accepted lifelong risk for all physicians. Physicians spend 10% of their career with at least one open medical malpractice claim.[45] Despite resident and attending concern about malpractice risk, education on legal issues is sorely underrepresented in medical school and residency curricula. Many EM residents enter the field with moderate malpractice concerns yet have little awareness of their actual risk and liability as residents.[3] This lack of knowledge, mixed with every physician's personal risk tolerance, leads to physician anxiety over risks associated with being held medically liable for adverse outcomes or care that is delivered by trainees under their supervision. These insecurities can prompt defensive medicine practices, thus increasing health care spending and inflating the cost of medical care.

Due to the lack of one comprehensive medical-legal database, current literature pulls from various imperfect federal, state, and insurer-generated databases. Based on the current data and the experience and recommendations of these authors, malpractice risk can be decreased with focused diagnostic testing, increased attention to high-risk pathologies, and increased resident supervision, especially regarding diagnostics, treatments, and procedures.

CLINICS CARE POINTS

- It is *not common* for an EM resident to be named in a malpractice case that results in payment (72% of claims do not result in indemnity)[2] or that reaches the public court system (94% of cases settle pre-court).[5]

- In the eyes of the law, a resident physician is held to the same standard of care as an attending physician in the same specialty.

- Issues with clinical judgment, communication, and documentation were differentiated as important contributing causes of malpractice risk.[9] Claims resulting in medical error were more likely to involve "excessive workloads, handoff issues, technical competence, and lack of supervision."[11]

- Attending supervision of residents is paramount. In many lawsuits involving residents, the basis for litigation is lack of adequate supervision.[7,10,17,18] In 2 studies of resident-centered litigation in EM, approximately one-fourth cases involved claims of inadequate supervision.[18,19]

- The most common reasons for which EM residents were named in malpractice cases involved diagnostic, treatment, and procedural errors.[7]

- Procedure-related complications were noted in 32% of resident malpractice cases, with vascular and spinal procedures being most common.[9]

- Highly reported areas of performance concerns included high-risk cardiovascular pathologies like acute myocardial infarction, pulmonary embolism, and cardiac arrest—the top 3 final diagnoses in EM malpractice claims (intubation as well as vascular and spinal procedures were other notable reported areas).[25] Knowing these areas are the highest contributors to claims will allow physicians to keep vigilant surrounding these risks.

- Good bedside manners expand to residents: Physicians who develop strong physician–patient trust relationships are less likely to be named in malpractice cases.[29]

DISCLOSURE

The opinions expressed in this article are solely the author's and do not represent the views of Troutman Pepper. This article is for informational purposes only and does not constitute legal advice. Please consult with a qualified legal professional for advice specific to your situation.

REFERENCES

1. Guardado JR. Policy Research Perspectives Medical Liability Claim Frequency Among U.S. Physicians. Available at: https://www.ama-assn.org/system/files/policy-research-perspective-medical-liability-claim-frequency.pdf. [Accessed 4 February 2024].

2. Mello MM, Chandra A, Gawande AA, et al. National costs of the medical liability system. Health Aff 2010;29(9):1569–77. https://doi.org/10.1377/hlthaff.2009.0807.

3. Rodriguez RM, Anglin D, Hankin A, et al. A Longitudinal Study of Emergency Medicine Residents' Malpractice Fear and Defensive Medicine. Acad Emerg Med 2007;14(6):569–73. https://doi.org/10.1197/j.aem.2007.01.020.

4. Department of Information Services/Applications and Data Analysis Accreditation Council for Graduate Medical Education. Data Resource Book Year 2022-2023. 2022nd-2023rd ed. Accreditation Council for Graduate Medical Education. 2023. Available at: https://www.acgme.org/globalassets/pfassets/publicationsbooks/2022-2023_acgme_databook_document.pdf. [Accessed 30 January 2024].

5. Glover M, McGee GW, Wilkinson DS, et al. Characteristics of Paid Malpractice Claims among Resident Physicians from 2001 to 2015 in the United States. Acad Med 2020;95(2):255–62. https://doi.org/10.1097/ACM.0000000000003039.

6. Wegman B, Stannard JP, Bal BS. Medical liability of the physician in training. Clin Orthop Relat Res 2012;470:1379–85. Springer New York LLC.

7. Poyorena C, Anderson A, Pollock JR, et al. A review of medical malpractice cases involving trainees in the emergency department. JACEP Open 2023;4(4). https://doi.org/10.1002/emp2.13014.

8. NPDB Guidebook. Chapter E: Reports, Reporting Medical Malpractice Payments. Available at: https://www.npdb.hrsa.gov/guidebook/EMMPR.jsp. [Accessed 29 January 2024].

9. Gurley KL, Grossman SA, Janes M, et al. Comparison of Emergency Medicine Malpractice Cases Involving Residents to Nonresident Cases. Acad Emerg Med 2018;25(9):980–6. https://doi.org/10.1111/acem.13430.

10. Myers LC, Gartland RM, Skillings J, et al. An examination of medical malpractice claims involving physician trainees. Acad Med 2020;95(8):1215–22. https://doi.org/10.1097/ACM.0000000000003117.

11. Singh H, Thomas EJ, Petersen LA, et al. Medical errors involving trainees: A study of closed malpractice claims from 5 insurers. Arch Intern Med 2007;167(19):2030–6.

12. Virshup BB. Strategic risk management: reducing malpractice claims through more effective patient-doctor communication. Am J Med Qual 1999;14(4):153–9.

13. Physician bedside manner linked to malpractice suit. Patient Focus Care 1997;5(5):58–9.

14. RDMJDVFR Levinson W. Physician-patient communication. The relationship with malpractice claims among primary care physicians and surgeons. JAMA 1997;277(7):553–9.

15. Supreme Court's Impact on Informed Consent Defenses. Marshall Dennehey. Available at: https://marshalldennehey.com/articles/supreme-court%E2%80%99s-impact-informed-consent-defenses. [Accessed 29 April 2024].

16. The Rise of Medical Battery and Informed Consent - TBA Law Blog. Available at: https://www.tba.org/index.cfm?pg=LawBlog&blAction=showEntry&blogEntry=25458. [Accessed 29 April 2024].

17. Nasca TJ, Day SH, Amis ES. The New Recommendations on Duty Hours from the ACGME Task Force. N Engl J Med 2010;363(2):e3. https://doi.org/10.1056/nejmsb1005800.
18. Antkowiak PS, Lai SY, Burke RC, et al. Characterizing malpractice cases involving emergency department advanced practice providers, physicians in training, and attending physicians. Acad Emerg Med 2023;30(12):1237–45. https://doi.org/10.1111/acem.14800.
19. Kachalia A, Gandhi TK, Puopolo AL, et al. Missed and Delayed Diagnoses in the Emergency Department: A Study of Closed Malpractice Claims From 4 Liability Insurers. Ann Emerg Med 2007;49(2):196–205. https://doi.org/10.1016/j.annemergmed.2006.06.035.
20. Snowdon DA, Hau R, Leggat SG, et al. Does clinical supervision of health professionals improve patient safety? A systematic review and meta-analysis. Int J Qual Health Care 2016;28(4):447–55. https://doi.org/10.1093/intqhc/mzw059.
21. Czeisler CA, Blum AB, Shea S, et al. Nature and Science of Sleep Dovepress Implementing the 2009 Institute of Medicine recommendations on resident physician work hours, supervision, and safety. Nat Sci Sleep 2011;3–47. https://doi.org/10.2147/NSS.S19649.
22. Jena AB, Seabury S, Lakdawalla D, et al. Malpractice Risk According to Physician Specialty. N Engl J Med 2011;365(7):629–36. https://doi.org/10.1056/NEJMSA1012370.
23. Richard Schauffler, Robert LaFountain, Shauna Strickland, et al. Examining the Work of State Courts: An Overview of 2015 State Court Caseloads. Available at: https://www.courtstatistics.org/__data/assets/pdf_file/0028/29818/2015-EWSC.pdf. [Accessed 4 February 2024].
24. Carrier ER, Reschovsky JD, Mello MM, et al. Physicians' fears of malpractice lawsuits are not assuaged by tort reforms. Health Aff (Millwood) 2010;29(9):1585–92. https://doi.org/10.1377/HLTHAFF.2010.0135.
25. Myers LC, Einbinder J, Camargo CA, et al. Characteristics of medical malpractice claims involving emergency medicine physicians. J Healthc Risk Manag 2021;41(1):9–15. https://doi.org/10.1002/JHRM.21450.
26. Centers for Medicare Services, Medicare Learning Network. MLN006347 – Guidelines for Teaching Physicians, Interns, & Residents. 2023. Available at: https://www.cms.gov/files/document/guidelines-teaching-physicians-interns-and-residents.pdf. [Accessed 4 February 2024].
27. Kilminster SM, Jolly BC. Effective supervision in clinical practice settings: A literature review. Med Educ 2000;34:827–40. https://doi.org/10.1046/j.1365-2923.2000.00758.x.
28. ACGME. ACGME Program Requirements for Graduate Medical Education in Emergency Medicine. Available at: www.acgme.org/OsteopathicRecognition.
29. Schleiter KE. HEALTH LAW Difficult Patient-Physician Relationships and the Risk of Medical Malpractice Litigation. 2009. Available at: www.virtualmentor.org.
30. Kachalia A, Kaufman SR, Boothman R, et al. Liability Claims and Costs Before and After Implementation of a Medical Error Disclosure Program. 2010. Available at: https://annals.org.
31. Gallagher TH, Studdert D, Levinson W. Disclosing Harmful Medical Errors to Patients. N Engl J Med 2007;356(26):2713–9. https://doi.org/10.1056/NEJMRA070568.
32. Berlin L, Berlin L. Will Saying "I'm Sorry" Prevent a Malpractice Lawsuit? AJR 2012;187(1):10–5. https://doi.org/10.2214/AJR.06.0110.

33. Updox Survey Reports 42 Percent of Americans Now Using Telehealth - Convenience (51%) and Speaking with Provider of Choice (49%) are Top Consumer Demands Post COVID-19. Available at: https://www.prweb.com/releases/updox-survey-reports-42-percent-of-americans-now-using-telehealth-convenience-51-and-speaking-with-provider-of-choice-49-are-top-consumer-demands-post-covid-19-848601637.html. [Accessed 23 January 2024].

34. Fogel AL, Kvedar JC. Reported Cases of Medical Malpractice in Direct-to-Consumer Telemedicine. JAMA 2019;321(13):1309. https://doi.org/10.1001/JAMA.2019.0395.

35. Noronha C, Lo MC, Nikiforova T, et al. Telehealth Competencies in Medical Education: New Frontiers in Faculty Development and Learner Assessments. J Gen Intern Med 2022;37(12):3168–73. https://doi.org/10.1007/s11606-022-07564-8.

36. Telehealth AAMC. Competencies Across the Learning Continuum. AAMC New and Emerging Areas in Medicine Series. Washington, DC: AAMC; 2021.

37. Medical Association A. HOD ACTION: Council on Medical Education Report 6 Adopted as Amended and the Remainder of the Report Filed. REPORT 6 OF THE COUNCIL ON MEDICAL EDUCATION (A-16) Telemedicine in Medical Education (Resolution 330-A-15) (Reference Committee C).; 2016.

38. Medical Association A. HOD ACTION: Council on Medical Education Report 6 adopted as amended and the remainder of the report filed. REPORT 6 OF THE COUNCIL ON MEDICAL EDUCATION (A-16) Telemedicine in Medical Education (Resolution 330-A-15) (Reference Committee C). Published online 2016.

39. ACGME. ACGME *Common Program Requirements*. Available at: https://www.acgme.org/globalassets/pfassets/programrequirements/cprresidency_2023.pdf. (Accessed 08 July 2024).

40. Direct Supervision Using Telecommunication Technology by Specialty Specialty-Specific Program Requirements: Available at: https://www.acgme.org/globalassets/pdfs/specialty-specific-requirement-topics/dio-direct_supervision_telecommunication.pdf. (Accessed 08 July 2024).

41. Centerfor Medicare Services, Medicare Learning Network M. MLN90175 - Telehealth Services. Available at: https://www.cms.gov/files/document/mln901705-telehealth-services.pdf. (Accessed 08 July 2024).

42. Center for Connected Health Policy. Center for Connected Health Policies. Available at: https://www.cchpca.org/all-telehealth-policies/. [Accessed 17 January 2024].

43. Telehealth.HHS.gov: Learn how to access or provide telehealth care. Available at: https://telehealth.hhs.gov/. [Accessed 27 January 2024].

44. Telehealth policy changes after the COVID-19 public health emergency | Telehealth.HHS.gov. Available at: https://telehealth.hhs.gov/providers/telehealth-policy/policy-changes-after-the-covid-19-public-health-emergency#temporary-medicare-changes-through-december-31,-2024. [Accessed 17 January 2024].

45. Seabury SA, Chandra A, Lakdawalla DN, et al. On average, physicians spend nearly 11 percent of their 40-year careers with an open, unresolved malpractice claim. Health Aff 2013;32(1):111–9. https://doi.org/10.1377/hlthaff.2012.0967.

Navigating Supervision of Advanced Practice Providers

Robert Rainer, MD, Kimberly Bambach, MD*

KEYWORDS

- Advanced practice provider • Nurse practitioner • Physician assistant
- Mid-level provider • Supervision • Billing • Documentation • Shared visit

KEY POINTS

- Current trends demonstrate that the proportion and complexity of emergency care provided by advanced practice providers (APPs) is increasing.
- Laws governing supervision vary between physician assistants and nurse practitioners, with the latter legally able to practice independently in some states.
- Supervision may be direct or indirect but contemporaneous with autonomy at the discretion of the emergency physician. Regardless of the supervision model, emergency medicine (EM) professional organizations advocate for physician-led teams.
- There are limited data on medicolegal risk in shared visits, but emergency physicians should be aware that they may be named in litigation if they are involved in a patient's care even if they did not have a face-to-face encounter.

INTRODUCTION AND CURRENT LANDSCAPE

Emergency care by physician assistants (PAs) and nurse practitioners (NPs) has increased dramatically in recent years. The emergency medicine (EM) workforce is comprised of 60% to 70% emergency physicians, 25% advanced practice providers (APPs-PAs and NPs collectively), and a small fraction of non-emergency physicians.[1] Similar numbers have been reported by other studies, which further delineated that PAs comprise 14.7% and NPs comprise 7.9% of the EM workforce.[2] From 2012 to 2018, the presence of APPs in the EM workforce has increased by 66%, with a 99% increase in NPs and 53% increase in PAs.[2] The number of US emergency departments (EDs) employing APPs has shown similar growth, with 28.3% of US EDs utilizing APPs in 1997, increasing to 77.2% by 2006.[3] Increased APP presence has been driven by an effort to decrease ED wait times, meet demand for low acuity visits, decrease costs, and combat the EM workforce shortage. This is particularly important in rural areas where access to care is limited.[3,4]

Department of Emergency Medicine, The Ohio State University, Columbus, OH, USA
* Corresponding author
E-mail address: Kimberly.bambach@osumc.edu

Emerg Med Clin N Am 43 (2025) 131–138
https://doi.org/10.1016/j.emc.2024.05.030
emed.theclinics.com
0733-8627/25/© 2024 Elsevier Inc. All rights are reserved, including those for text and data mining, AI training, and similar technologies.

APPs are regarded as valuable members of the EM workforce, but there has been controversy surrounding APP scope of practice and the increasing number of visits where an APP was the sole clinician involved in a patient's care (ie, independent practice or "APP only" visits). There has been a marked increase in the number of ED patients seen independently by APPs; as of 1995, these comprised only 1.1% of all ED visits, progressing to 14.3% in 2019.[4-6] While the overall patient population is becoming increasingly complex, APPs provide an increasing proportion of high acuity care. From 2013 to 2019, the percentage of rural high acuity ED visits billed independently by APPs increased from 7.3% to 16.4%; during this time frame, rural emergency physicians had a 14.4% increase in overall high acuity billing while APPs experienced a 58.8% increase.[6] While this is more pronounced in rural areas, where APPs see a larger proportion of ED visits due to emergency physician staffing shortages, this has also been shown in urban settings, where the percentage of high acuity ED visits billed independently by APPs increased from 4.8% to 8.8% during the same time frame.[6] An influential 2021 EM workforce projection predicted an oversupply of emergency physicians in 2030. Increasing integration of APPs in emergency care contributed to these projections, with APPs expected to manage up to 20% of ED visits by 2030.[2] The changing landscape of the EM workforce was also a factor in the unexpected 2023 EM match results, with 554 initially unfilled residency positions.[7]

This changing practice landscape underscores the importance of understanding key elements related to the emergency physician's supervisory role. While 75% of program directors agreed that residents should learn how to work with an interdisciplinary team, 49% reported no dedicated curricular time to the supervision of and collaboration with APPs and only 15% reported that residents supervise APPs as part of their training.[8] Carpenter and colleagues and the American College of Emergency Physicians (ACEP) both recommend that all programs should provide residents with the opportunity to supervise APPs clinically and should dedicate curricular time to interprofessional team training.[8,9] In this article, we will discuss an approach to APP supervision in depth to equip emergency physicians with the skillset to both effectively navigate interprofessional dynamics and mitigate medicolegal risk.

LAWS AND GUIDELINES OF ADVANCED PRACTICE PROVIDER SUPERVISION

The legal practice authority of NPs and PA differs significantly. In all states, PAs are required to work under a supervisory physician and do not practice independently, although supervision may be direct or indirect. In most states, PA licensure is regulated by the state's medical board. The number of PAs that a physician may supervise is also limited, between 4 and 6 at any given time. In contrast, NP scope of practice varies by state and some NPs may legally practice without physician oversight with licensure regulated by state nursing boards. In 27 states and Washington D.C., the American Association of Nurse Practitioners (AANP) characterizes the practice environment as "full practice" which means that NPs prescribe, diagnose, and treat patients without physician supervision. In 12 states, the practice environment is considered "reduced" which means at least one aspect of NP practice is limited and NPs may collaborate with a physician. In 11 states with "restricted" NP practice, physicians provide career-long supervision.[10] There has been a significant drive from NP advocacy groups for independent practice.[11-13]

While recognizing that APPs are integral and valued team members, the American Medical Association and all major EM professional organizations including the ACEP and the American Academy of Emergency Medicine advocate for ED teams to be physician-led.[9,14,15] In 2023, ACEP updated a policy guideline stating that PAs and NPs should not perform independent, unsupervised care in the ED.[9]

FACTORS AFFECTING SUPERVISION AND SCOPE OF PRACTICE

In general, there is little standardization regarding APP supervision and scope of practice and this often varies by state and federal regulations, facility/institutional policies, education and experience, and supervising physician delegation.[16] In nearly all states, APP scope of practice is determined by the scope of practice of the supervising physician. There is an important distinction between regulatory and operational supervision. Regulatory supervision refers to oversight that is mandated by regulatory bodies, such as requirements by the Centers for Medicare and Medicaid Services for billing or state laws, while operational supervision refers to the model of oversight implemented by a given ED that is inherently variable by state, site, or institution.[13]

Models—Direct Versus Indirect Supervision

There are several models of supervision. Supervision may be direct, meaning that the supervising emergency physician personally examines and evaluates the patient, which is the gold standard of supervision. Supervision may also be indirect, at the discretion of the supervising physician, which includes contemporaneously discussing or reviewing the management of the patient even if they do not personally evaluate the patient.

Supervision may also be further broken down by the location of the supervising emergency physician. The supervising physician may be onsite, or physically present in the ED and available to evaluate a patient, as opposed to offsite and not physically present in the ED but available for discussion of patient management. *It is important to note that chart review in a non-contemporaneous manner does not constitute direct or indirect supervision*, and is not considered to be an acceptable model of supervision by ACEP, which states that emergency physicians should not be required to sign the chart of a patient unless they have a real-time opportunity to be involved in the patient's care.[9] The Society of Emergency Medicine PAs (SEMPA) also agrees that emergency physicians should not be required to co-sign charts unless they were directly involved in a patient's care.[17]

Despite ACEP guidelines, this is largely state and site dependent and supervision lacks a clear unifying definition. Most states require that an APPs work must be reviewed at some point and that a physician should be available for consultation if needed. However, few regulations exist to delineate direct or indirect supervision, onsite or offsite supervision, level of patient or procedural complexity that merits supervision, or limitations on asynchronous chart review. Supervisory policies should be understood by the emergency physician when accepting a new position or signing a contract.

Acuity—the Impact of Emergency Severity Index on Advanced Practice Provider Supervision

Higher acuity, often represented by lower Emergency Severity Index (ESI) level, is typically associated with an increased level of supervision. In fact, 53.7% of EDs do not consider caring for ESI Level 1 patients to be within the APP scope of practice.[18] However, this too is highly variable and site dependent, and of the EDs that do consider this to be within the APP scope of practice, 10% do not require the emergency physician to be notified. Conversely, indirect supervision or independent evaluation of lower acuity (ie, ESI Levels 4–5) is fairly commonplace. However, as previously discussed, the overall acuity of emergency care is increasing and APPs are providing more complex care with decreased oversight.[6]

Practice Setting—Workforce Limitations in Rural Locations

The ACEP policy statement acknowledges the current workforce limitations related to rural emergency care, such as the need for access to a supervising physician via telehealth for critical access and rural EDs. The use of indirect offsite supervisory models is approved for use in Critical Access Hospitals and Rural Emergency Hospitals, with the understanding that an emergency physician is available at all times for real-time discussion of patient management.[9] Supervision is typically greater in academic and urban sites as opposed to community or rural hospitals[19] whereas independent practice is more prevalent in rural settings.[6]

Education and Experience of Physician Assistants and Nurse Practitioners

Given the variability of APP education and experience, emergency physicians should familiarize themselves with the basic requirements for APP training/education as well as the specific education and experience of the APP under supervision. The differences between PA and NP education do not result in significant scope of practice differences in the ED.[13] It has been shown that an emergency physician's familiarity with a given APPs competence and medical decision making (MDM) will affect the level of supervision and scope of practice, with increased personal experience and trust allowing for greater scope of practice and decreased oversight. Specific roles and privileges, including procedural performance, are typically determined on an institutional or site-specific basis.[2,16]

1. Physician Assistant (PA)

PAs must graduate from master's programs accredited by the Accreditation Review Commission for Educations of Physician Assistants. These programs range from 24 to 26 months in duration and involve at least 12 months of clinical rotations in internal medicine, family medicine, surgery, pediatrics, obstetrics and gynecology, EM, and behavioral and mental health. Clinical experience requirements for PA school applicants vary from 2000 hours to "experience preferred," but admitted applicants have an average of 3500 hours of health care experience prior to matriculation. Some EM specific PA training programs exist, which involve an additional 12 to 18 months with rotations in EM, critical care, ultrasound, and trauma. However, these programs are not required for PAs to practice in EDs and as of 2017, only 11% of PAs that practice EM had completed such a program.[12,16]

2. Nurse Practitioner (NP)

There are 4 types of Advanced Practice Registered Nurses, including Certified Registered Nurse Anesthetists, Certified Nurse Midwifes, Clinical Nurse Specialists, and Certified Nurse Practitioners (CNP). CNPs are capable of practicing in EDs. NP Programs are accredited by the Commission on Collegiate Nursing Education and include both Masters of Science in Nursing and Doctorate of Nursing Practice programs. Master's programs require 500 hours of post-bachelors training and doctoral programs require 1000 hours of post-baccalaureate training. Training is based on a specific population focus and includes family, adult/gerontology, pediatrics, psychiatry, and women's health. The majority of EM NPs choose a family population focus, as this enables them to care for all ages including pediatric patients. However, some NPs may choose an adult/gerontology population focus as this provides the opportunity for an acute care nursing specialization, but this limits scope of practice to patients greater than 12 year old. NP program applicants typically have a Bachelor of Science in Nursing. The majority of NP programs require 1 to 2 years, or 2000 to 4000 hours, of nursing experience prior to matriculation. However, there has been an increase in direct-entry NP programs, which allow for entry without any bedside nursing experience. There are some post-graduate programs that focus specifically on EM, which provide additional clinical time in ED or urgent care settings; however, these are not required to practice in an ED.[12,16]

CODING, BILLING, AND DOCUMENTATION

In 2023, CMS updated the Evaluation and Management (E/M) services guide, which made major changes to EM billing and coding.[20] These changes were the first substantial changes in several decades and have key implications for supervised visits. A "shared visit" is defined as a physician and an APP in the same group that each personally performs a part of a visit. Revised guidelines for 2024 state that the physician or APP who provides greater than 50% of the total time spent with the patient or a substantive part of the MDM should bill for the visit. If the emergency physician provides a substantive part of the MDM, they may bill for the encounter even if the APP is the sole clinician to perform a face-to-face evaluation. APPs may also bill for critical care time. Critical care time provided by the ED physician and APP may be summed, but it may only be submitted once by the individual who performed greater than 50% of the critical care time.[21] APPs may bill for services at 85% of the Medicare Physician Fee. Procedures, however, cannot be shared and if performed by an APP are also billed at 85%. It is not sufficient to document that one simply agrees with or attests to the APPs plan for medical care. One example for documentation that would qualify to be coded appropriately to bill care by an emergency physician may be: "I saw and evaluated the patient with the APP. I personally performed the MDM for this encounter and provided a substantive portion of care. I discussed the patient with neurology. They recommended MRI brain with and without contrast. We will admit the patient for further care."

MEDICOLEGAL AND RISK MITIGATION

There are unfortunately limited data available regarding the medicolegal risks and implications of continued expansion of APP presence in US EDs. However, it is clear that throughout all specialties, there has been an increase in malpractice claims involving a PA or NP, with increases noted yearly between 2005 and 2015.[22] Antkowiak and colleagues specifically focused on malpractice cases in EM and sought to delineate factors contributing to the medicolegal risk associated with the increased presence of APPs. Of the EM malpractice claims examined between 2010 and 2019, 3.3% involved an NP, 8.8% involved a PA, and 78% involved an attending physician only. APP cases also resulted in a greater average gross indemnity paid compared to no-extender cases. Regarding malpractice claims involving APPs, clinical judgment, documentation, and supervision were more commonly noted to be contributing factors compared to no-extender cases.[23]

Although there are limited data on medicolegal risk in shared visits, emergency physicians should be aware that they may be named in litigation if they are involved in a patient's care even if they did not have a face-to-face encounter. The supervisory role of emergency physicians is a main medicolegal focus, as lack of sufficient oversight and standardization of supervisory models are strongly believed to contribute to malpractice risk. Regardless of the supervisory model used, the emergency physician is often named as a co-defendant in malpractice claims. While legal proceedings may take into account institutional or state-specific policies limiting physician liability, this should not be relied on as a point of safety.[13] Emergency physicians should be mindful of the potential for high-risk diagnoses, even if the patient is evaluated by an APP in a low acuity "fast track" area of the ED. Chief complaints of chest pain (missed acute myocardial infarction), abdominal pain (missed appendicitis, missed abdominal aortic aneurysm), pediatric fever (missed meningitis), and lacerations with neurovascular or motor compromise (missed tendon injuries) should prompt additional oversight by the emergency physician. A higher rate of diagnosis-related errors by APPs compared to physicians has been reported in literature that is not specific to EM.[22]

Documentation is frequently scrutinized when legal action is pursued, and inconsistent documentation is a source of medicolegal risk. If there is a discrepancy between APP and physician documentation, it should be addressed in the physician's documentation. Physicians should carefully document their own independent findings and MDM. Failure to review family history, lack of documentation of the MDM, and weak documentation of reassessment prior to discharge are key sources of risk.[24] Supervising emergency physicians should educate collaborating APPs on key protective practices of documentation. These practices include:

1. Clear documentation of MDM, particularly when there is diagnostic uncertainty or a high-risk chief complaint.
2. Follow-up of results.
3. Robust documentation of reassessment prior to discharge.
4. Broad categories used to document clinical impressions which acknowledge alternative diagnoses (such as a discharge of abdominal pain rather than acute gastroenteritis, as the patient may have early appendicitis).
5. Providing and documenting return precautions and a follow-up plan.[25]

These principles all demonstrate how communication with APP colleagues is critical in shared visits.

SUMMARY

Current workforce trends demonstrate that the proportion and complexity of emergency care provided by APPs is increasing, which underscores the importance of emergency physician supervision and support. PAs always work with a supervising physician, while NPs may legally practice independently in some states. Many factors affect APP supervision and scope of practice including the supervision model, practice setting and site-specific policies, patient acuity, APP education and training, and APP experience. Emergency physicians should be aware that ACEP does not support non-contemporaneous chart review as a supervision model and they should be mindful of chart review expectations when reviewing new contracts to avoid this source of risk. Emergency physicians can mitigate risk by effective communication, attention to high risk diagnoses, and sound documentation practices.

CLINICS CARE POINTS

- Asynchronous chart review is not considered by the American College of Emergency Physicians to be appropriate oversight.
- 2023 Evaluation and Management (E/M) Guidelines changed coding, billing, and by extension documentation, substantially. EM physicians may bill for care when they spend

greater than 50% of the time caring for the patient or a substantive portion of the medical decision making.
• Communication lapses and contradictory documentation with errors and omissions are potential sources of medical error and risk. Ensuring appropriate oversight with consideration of the APPs experience and documentation may minimize legal risk.

DISCLOSURE

The authors have no financial disclosures.

REFERENCES

1. Kennedy HM, Burns K, Carius M, et al. State of the National Emergency Department Workforce: Who Provides Care Where? Ann Emerg Med 2018;72(3):302–7.
2. Marco CA, Mark Courtney D, Ling LJ, et al. The emergency medicine physician workforce: projections for 2030. Ann Emerg Med 2021;78(6):726–37.
3. Menchine MD, Wiechmann W, Rudkin S. Trends in midlevel provider utilization in emergency departments from 1997 to 2006. Acad Emerg Med 2009;16(10): 963–9.
4. Wiler JL, Rooks SP, Ginde AA. Update on midlevel provider utilization in U.S. emergency departments, 2006 to 2009. Acad Emerg Med 2012;19(8):986–9.
5. Brown DFM, Sullivan AF, Espinola JA, et al. Continued rise in the use of mid-level providers in US emergency departments, 1993–2009. Int J Emerg Med 2012; 5(1):21.
6. Gettel CJ, Schuur JD, Mullen JB, et al. Rising high-acuity emergency care services independently billed by advanced practice providers, 2013 to 2019. Acad Emerg Med 2023;30:89–98.
7. Bennett CL, Lin M, Camargo CA. Challenges surrounding the emergency physician workforce and their impact on the emergency medicine match. Clin Exp Emerg Med 2023;10(4):349–53.
8. Carpenter CR, Abrams S, Mark Courtney D, et al. Advanced practice providers in academic emergency medicine: a national survey of chairs and program directors. Acad Emerg Med 2021;29:184–92.
9. American College of Emergency Physicians. Guidelines Regarding the Role of Physician Assistants and Nurse Practitioners in the Emergency Department. Available at: www.acep.org/siteassets/new-pdfs/policy-statements/guidelines-reg-the-role-of-physician-assistants-and-nurse-practitioners-in-the-ed.pdf://www.acep.org/siteassets/new-pdfs/policy-statements/guidelines-reg-the-role-of-physician-assistants-and-nurse-practitioners-in-the-ed.pdf. (Accessed 25 July 2024).
10. American Association of Nurse Practitioners. State practice environment. 2023. Available at: https://www.aanp.org/advocacy/state/state-practice-environment. [Accessed 27 January 2024].
11. Thomas S. Open letter to the AMA, AAEM and AAEM/RSA. American Association Of Nurse Practitioners. 2019. Available at: https://www.aanp.org/news-feed/open-letter-to-the-ama-aaem-and-aaem-rsa. [Accessed 23 January 2024].
12. Chekijian SA, Elia TR, Horton JL, et al. A Review of interprofessional variation in education: challenges and considerations in the growth of advanced practice providers in emergency medicine. AEM Educ Train 2021;5:1–10.
13. Klauer K. Innovative staffing in emergency departments: the role of midlevel providers. CJEM 2013;15(3):134–40.

14. American College of Emergency Physicians. Joint statement regarding post-graduate training of nurse practitioners and physician assistants. 2020. Available at: https://www.acep.org/administration/personnel-team-management/post-graduate-training-of-nps-and-pas. [Accessed 4 March 2024].

15. American Academy of Emergency Medicine. Updated position statement on non-physician practitioners. american academy of emergency medicine. 2020. Available at: https://www.aaem.org/statements/updated-position-statement-on-non-physician-practitioners/. [Accessed 23 January 2024].

16. Katz J, Powers M, Amusina O. A review of procedural skills performed by advanced practice providers in emergency department and critical care settings. Dis Mon 2021;67:101013.

17. Society of Emergency Medicine Physician Assistants. SEMPA statement regarding AAEM's Policy on APPs.; 2019. Available at: https://sempa.org/wp-content/uploads/2023/12/sempa-statement-regarding-aaems-app-policy-febraury-8-20191.pdf. (Accessed 25 July 2024).

18. Phillips AW, Klauer KM, Kessler CS. Emergency physician evaluation of PA and NP practice patterns. J Am Acad Physician Assist 2018;31(5):38–43.

19. Chekijian SA, Elia TR, Monti JE, et al. Integration of advanced practice providers in academic emergency departments: best practices and considerations. AEM Educ Train 2018;2(S1):S48–55.

20. Evaluation and Management Services Guide. In: Medicare learning network booklet. ; 2023:1-21.Available at: https://www.cms.gov/outreach-and-education/medicare-learning-network-mln/mlnproducts/downloads/eval-mgmt-serv-guide-icn006764.pdf. (Accessed 25 July 2024).

21. American College of Emergency Physicians. Shared Services. 2023. Available at: https://www.acep.org/administration/reimbursement/reimbursement-faqs/Shared-Services-FAQ. [Accessed 4 March 2024].

22. Brock DM, Nicholson JG, Hooker RS. Physician assistant and nurse practitioner malpractice trends. Med Care Res Rev 2016;74(5):613–24.

23. Antkowiak PS, Lai S-Y, Burke RC, et al. Characterizing malpractice cases involving emergency department advanced practice providers, physicians in training, and attending physicians. Acad Emerg Med 2023;30:1237–45.

24. Bergen J.M., MACEP risk management course: module 8: practice environment. In: Massachusetts College of Emergency Physicians. ; 2016. Available at: https://nuhem.com/wp-content/uploads/2021/06/8-Risk-Management.pdf. (Accessed 25 July 2024).

25. Ghaith S, Moore GP, Colbenson KM, et al. Charting practices to protect against malpractice: case reviews and learning points. West J Emerg Med 2022;23(3):412–7.

Understanding Against Medical Advice, Informed Consent, and Emergency Medical Treatment and Labor Act

Fernanda Calienes Cerpa, MD, PGY2[a],*,
Stephen Anthony Colucciello, MD[b]

KEYWORDS

- EMTALA • AMA • Informed consent • Shared decision-making
- Emergency medical condition • Medical screening examination

KEY POINTS

- Left without treatment being completed: some patients who leave without being seen or before treatment is complete may have higher acuity complaints. A physician should review these charts to determine if further action is necessary (such as contacting the patient via telephone).
- Against medical advice: this is a process and not simply a signature. Talk to the patient and determine why they want to leave, explore alternative approaches, use shared decision-making, assess decision-making capacity, and document well.
- EMTALA: perform a timely medical screening exam, always stabilize within constraints of your hospital, transfer to higher level of care when benefits outweigh the risks, always err on the side of what is best for the patient. Document well.
- Informed consent: this includes disclosing the condition being treated, the proposed treatment or procedure, anticipated results of the proposed plan, the practical alternative treatments including non-treatment, and recognizing the risks and benefits involved. It is crucial to determine decision-making capacity.

The emergency department (ED) is a fast-paced environment. A framework for approaching daily events, such as when patients leave prior to receiving the recommended examination or treatment, is important for patient safety and to protect against litigation. We will discuss frequent questions, strategies, and myths regarding discharges against medical advice (AMA; **Fig. 1**).

[a] Emergency Department, Carolinas Medical Center, 1000 Blythe Boulevard, Charlotte, NC 28203, USA; [b] Emergency Medicine Carolinas Medical Center/Wake Forest Medical School, 1000 Blythe Boulevard, Charlotte, NC 28203, USA
* Corresponding author. 1000 Blythe Boulevard, Charlotte, NC 28203.
E-mail address: fernanda.calienescerpa@atriumhealth.org
Twitter: @CalienesMD (S.A.C.)

Emerg Med Clin N Am 43 (2025) 139–154
https://doi.org/10.1016/j.emc.2024.05.022
0733-8627/25/© 2024 Elsevier Inc. All rights are reserved, including those for text and data mining, AI training, and similar technologies.

Left Without Being Seen (LWBS)	Left Before Treatment Completed (LBTC)	Left Against Medical Advice (AMA)
The first occurs when the patient leaves prior to initiation of a medical screening examination. For example, the patient checks in to the ED, but leaves before a provider conducts an examination or obtains a history.	The second is when the patient leaves the ED when workup has been initiated, but test results are not known or communicated to the patient.	The final situation is when the physician has been able to interact with the patient and have a meaningful conversation, but the patient declines further care.

Fig. 1. Three scenarios in which a patient leaves the emergency department "early."

LEFT WITHOUT BEING SEEN

Contrary to what many emergency providers think, up to 30% of patients who leave without being seen have higher acuity chief complaints.[1] They also have nearly triple the number of ED visits as the general ED patient.[2] Lower odds for left without being seen (LWBS) are associated with age less than 18 years, greater than 65 years, zip codes with higher median quartiles, chronic condition, weekend presentations, and Medicare, Tricare, Workman's Compensation, or private insurance.[3] LWBS rates are disproportionately higher in low-income and poorly insured patients.[4]

The primary reason for leaving is long wait times. Wait times vary widely by state, peak days, and hospital expected annual volume. From 2016 data, the average wait time for ED treatment is 24.1 minutes in EDs with less than 20,000 annual visits, 34.5 minutes in EDs with 20,000 to 49,999 annual visits, and 48.7 minutes in EDs with 50,000 or more annual visits.[5] These wait times vary widely by state. From the latest National Center for Health Statistics data from 2021 using 139,781 visits, the median wait time to see a physician, advanced practice registered nurse, or physician assistant was 37.5 minutes. About 3% of all ED visits had a wait time of 3 or more hours.[6] Furthermore, over half of LWBS cases seek medical attention within 1 week, but there are cases that require hospitalizations, urgent surgery, and occasionally patients die after LWBS.

The challenging aspect is that there are few simple (or inexpensive) methods of improving wait times and a multitude of compounding factors. Wait times are impacted by ED boarding, bed availability, physical space, admission/discharge rates, staffing, resources, ED volume, admitting procedures, efficiency, and multiple other bottlenecks in the health care system.

Historically, administrators considered LWBS numbers as a management issue rather than a system-level concern. Most administrators now realize that LWBS numbers may be a "canary in the coal mine" for a stressed ED. Solutions to counteract this issue often rely on fixes to mitigate ED crowding with varying levels of success. Some of these examples include provider-in-triage, implementing vital signs booths, split-flow models to provide more rapid screening, and using predictive analytics for variable staffing models.[7] Other strategies include telemedicine for triage surges or calling in additional personnel when door-to-provider time exceeds a predetermined metric. In a study by Sember and colleagues, adding a provider in triage at St. Elizabeth Youngstown Hospital, a level 1 trauma center, decreased LWBS rate from 5% to 1%.[8] Split-flow models help identify and separate high-acuity and low-acuity patients to streamline care. A "vertical split flow" model is when existing ED space is created by removing horizontal stretchers and replacing them with multiple chairs to allow assessment and management in an upright sitting position. So only "horizontal" patients who must remain recumbent get placed in a room on a stretcher while "vertical" patients who can sit in a chair are clustered in a common area. In a 2023 study incorporating 10,638 patient visits, vertical split flow models reduced overall length of stay and improved throughput for emergency severity index (ESI) level 3 patients.[9] Although these are encouraging studies, focusing on one metric in isolation may lead to unintended consequences. For example, meeting the needs of the many can overwhelm providers and compromise the quality of care for both the ambulatory patients and the critically ill.

Many emergency departments will list a patient as LWBS once 3 attempts to locate the patient are documented. These authors recommend consideration for the following approach with modifications as indicated by circumstance (**Fig. 2**).

Certain hospitals have also implemented the use of beeper/paging systems such as a pager to alert patients when they can be seen by a provider. Theoretically, it allows some mobility and freedom of choice while they wait. This system was studied in a pediatric emergency department by Scolnik and colleagues, which was viewed favorably by patients, but did not impact satisfaction scores.[10]

LEFT BEFORE TREATMENT COMPLETE

A multicenter retrospective study by Smalley and colleagues found that most (2812 patients) who left before treatment were completed returned within less than 24 hours, with 76.1% returning in 10 days. Of those that returned, 23.2% were admitted.[11]

Following the 21st Century Cures Act, a federal law requiring the immediate electronic availability of test results to patients, it is unclear if more patients now leave without speaking to the provider once they know their results of laboratories and/or imaging. This can be a safety concern as laboratories need to be interpreted in the context of the ED presentation and sometimes require intervention. Failure to follow up on results not communicated or explained to patients can lead to missed or delayed diagnosis and have medico-legal implications. Each emergency department needs a well-implemented mechanism to follow up on test results that return after patients leave the ED.

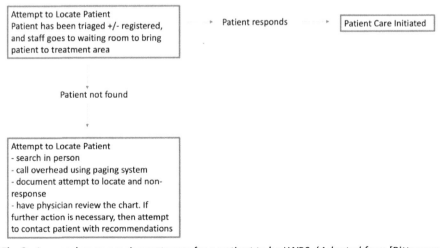

Fig. 2. Approaches as per circumstances for a patient to be LWBS. (*Adapted from* [Bitterman R MD, JD, FACEP. Against Medical Advice (AMA). *EPIX PRINCIPLES.* November 2011]; with permission needing to include.)

AGAINST MEDICAL ADVICE: A *PROCESS* AND NOT SIMPLY A SIGNATURE

This section will discuss relevant definitions, unique challenges of informed consent in the emergency department, and help prepare medical providers for how to approach complex patient encounters with the goal of maximizing benefit.

AMA is a term used when a patient chooses to leave the hospital before a treating physician recommends discharge. Although it may appear to be conceptually straight-forward, there are multiple considerations that are frequently ignored. Providers must respect the patient's self-determination, communicate concerns effectively, and prop-erly document events. Providers must understand the process of informed consent and, to "the best of your ability and judgment," include issues relevant to the practical management of AMA discharges. The AMA encounter can be a frustrating issue for both physicians and patients; however, patients with decision-making capacity are entitled to decline any recommended treatment. *Emergency providers must always remember that AMA is a process and not simply a signature.*

In a report published in 2012 by the Healthcare Cost and Utilization Project, there was a 41% increase in AMA discharges between 1997 and 2011. Every year United States has about 500,000 patients requesting to leave AMA.[12] Choi and colleagues, in a retrospective study of 656 patients, found that those who left AMA had a risk of readmission 12 times higher compared to non-AMA groups and an increased 12 month all-cause mortality.[13]

Categorized into 4 distinct categories, the following factors increase the likelihood of patients leaving AMA (**Fig. 3**).

There is a paucity of studies that adequately address disparities in AMA discharges and how they affect minority patients or patients of color. In a study sample of 33,147,251 ED visits to 989 hospitals, 1.6% of visits resulted in leaving AMA; rates were higher for Black patients (2.1%) compared with Hispanic (1.6%) and White (1.4%) patients. However, after adjusting for each hospital's baseline AMA rate and patient sociodemographic factors, Black and Hispanic patients had lower odds of leaving AMA compared to White patients. This change was dependent on hospital location and the baseline number of patients of color seen/treated rather than patient characteristics. This study calculated that if ED care of Black patients were distributed evenly across hospitals in the United States rather than more concentrated in a small number of hospitals with high AMA rates, there would be 217,544 fewer AMAs in the Black patient population per year.[14]

Efforts to reduce racial and ethnic disparities in AMA rates should prioritize interven-tions aimed at addressing medical segregation and equitable distribution of re-sources. These are not easy tasks and are beyond this study's scope.

AGAINST MEDICAL ADVICE FRAMEWORK

As an emergency medicine provider, having a step-by-step framework is helpful both for yourself and for patients leaving AMA.

1. Patient-centered approach
   - Seek why the patient wants to leave AMA
   - Avoid judgment, assuming, or stigmatizing the patient
     - "Do not take the AMA personally or get defensive"
   - Address the patient's concerns and needs
   - Think of a multidisciplinary approach and support
     - Consider involving family, friends, or the primary care provider (PCP) in the decision-making process (with permission of the patient)

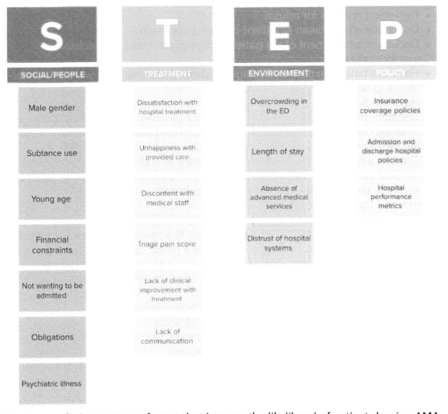

Fig. 3. Four distinct category factors that increase the likelihood of patients leaving AMA. (*Adapted from* [Albayati A. Why Do Patients Leave against Medical Advice? Reasons, Consequences, Prevention, and Interventions. NIH. https://www.ncbi.nlm.nih.gov/pmc/articles/PMC7909809/. Published January 21, 2021. Accessed January 30, 2024]; with permission needing to include.)

2. Alternative plan and harm reduction
   - Remember that a suboptimal plan is better than no plan
   - Support the patient's treatment goals
   - Identify barriers and resolve them if able
   - Provide prescriptions and follow-up care
     - Many providers mistakenly believe that medicines should not or cannot be prescribed to an AMA patient
   - Ensure the patient understands they can return at any time if needed
     - Put this in the discharge instructions
   - Go over discharge instructions including reasons to return
3. Informed refusal
   - Discuss your working or actual diagnosis/findings
   - Discuss recommended course of treatment including alternatives
   - Discuss comfort measures if applicable
   - Discuss risk of refusing treatment
4. Documentation
   - Document treatment(s) offered, risk/benefits of further treatment and no treatment

- Document reasons for refusal
- Document efforts taken at patient-centered approach
- Document assessment of the patient's capacity to make the decision
5. Capacity evaluation
   - Have the patient explain their diagnosis/findings in their own words ("I understand" is not enough)
   - Have the patient explain the consequences of leaving AMA
   - Capacity determination is made by an ED clinician or eligible psychologist, whereas competence is made by the courts. If the patient does not have capacity, then continue patient care and locate a surrogate decision-maker
   - There is a hierarchy (that may differ from state to state) for who can consent to medical treatment on behalf of a patient who is comatose or otherwise lacks capacity to communicate their health care decisions:
   - In North Carolina the hierarchical order is:
     - The legal guardian of the patient including one appointed by a court
     - The health care agent appointed pursuant to a health care power of attorney
     - An agent appointed by the patient to make health care decisions
     - The patient's spouse
     - Available children who are aged at least 18 years who demonstrate decision-making capacity
     - Available parents who demonstrate decision-making capacity
     - Available siblings who are aged at least 18 years
     - An individual in a relationship with the patient who is acting in good faith on behalf of patient and can convey their wishes
     - If the persons listed earlier are not available, then the attending physician at their discretion may provide consent. It is best to obtain written confirmation by a second physician. However, confirmation should never delay care if it would endanger the life of the patient

EXAMPLE OF AGAINST MEDICAL ADVICE ADDENDUM

The patient presented with a chief complaint of ___ and has expressed the desire to leave AMA. Based on history, physical examination, and studies returned to date, I have explained my concern that ___. I have explained my recommendation for ___ and offered alternative treatment options that include ___. I also explained that leaving places them at risk for worsening condition, critical illness, death, temporary or permanent disability including ___. Their reasons for leaving AMA are due to ___. To resolve reasons for leaving, I have ___. I ensured there were no communications barriers by ___.

The patient is clinically sober, without injury to affect their cognition, has intact insight, judgment, reasoning, and demonstrates the capacity to make their own health care decisions. Despite efforts, the patient was unwilling to stay. Harm reduction strategies such as ____ (ie, prescriptions, specialty or PCP follow-up) was provided to help increase the probability of a good outcome. I repeated that they may return to the emergency department for additional testing and care at any time. This conversation was witnessed by ___. AMA paperwork was ___ completed and signed.

COMMON MYTHS OF AGAINST MEDICAL ADVICE
If a Patient Leaves Against Medical Advice, Then Their Insurance Will not Cover the Visit

According to a survey published in the Journal of General Internal Medicine, close to two-thirds of residents and almost half of attending physicians believe that leaving

AMA will force the patient to cover the full hospital bill. This is a misconception. The threat of financial penalties should not be used as a threat or "leverage" technique to persuade a patient to stay. For example, in a study of 46,319 patients during a 9 year period, among those insured, payment was refused in 4.1% of cases; however, no cases were because of leaving AMA.[15] The most common reason for payment refusal was an administrative issue such as an incorrect or misspelled name.

The Patient that Left Against Medical Advice Is a "Problem" Patient

It is easy to link AMA to those situations where someone was frustrated, angry, or agitated with the care provided. The reality is that there are broad and complex reasons that influence a patient's decision to leave AMA. These may include work, family or pet care obligations, unrealistic expectations, short staffing, resource limitations, degree of risk aversion of the patient and the physician, as well as the physician's bedside manner.

Having the Patient Sign the Against Medical Advice Form Gets You Off the Hook

Signing this form does not have a significant legal protection on its own (although it should be requested). Since courts do not view a signed form as a complete waiver of liability, if there was a "one or the other" situation, the documentation of the encounter including capacity and risks is most important, but the form should also be signed when patients leave AMA.

Once the Patient Decides to Leave Against Medical Advice, Your Duty as a Physician Is Done

False. Once this decision has been made, one must ensure that this discharge is as safe as possible under the circumstances, including recommendations for outpatient care and prescriptions.

INFORMED CONSENT

Informed consent laws first began at the beginning of the twentieth century. Justice Benjamin Cardozo's response to a landmark case, Mary Schloendorff v Society of New York Hospital in 1914, helped establish the legal basis of consent. The Schloendorff case involved an unauthorized surgery on an anesthetized patient with a fibroid tumor. This surgery was done to better visualize but not to remove the mass. Following this operation, the patient developed gangrene to her fingers, which required amputation. Cardozo wrote, "Every human being of adult years and sound mind has a right to determine what shall be done with his own body; and a surgeon who performs an operation without his patient's consent commits an assault for which he is liable in damages."[16] In this case, the court found the plaintiff did not consent and thus a victim of medical battery. The ethical principle of Cardozo's words still guides medical behavior. Other famous cases further defined the meaning of informed consent.

Canterbury v Spence, identified key pieces of information that a physician must disclose including

- The condition being treated
- The nature and character of the proposed treatment or surgical procedure
- The anticipated results from the proposed treatment or surgical procedure
- The recognized practical alternative forms of treatment including nontreatment
- The recognized serious risks, complications, and anticipated benefits involved in the treatment or surgical procedure.[17]

In Gates v Jensen (1979), the Washington State Supreme Court held that a physician has a duty to inform a patient of abnormalities, in this case, relating to elevated ocular pressures. Jandre v Physicians Insurance Co. of Wisconsin clarified the issue of "reasonable patient standard," which states that "a doctor must provide the patient with the information a reasonable person in the patients position would regard as significant when deciding to accept or reject a diagnostic procedure."[18] Similarly, the decision in Nixdorf v Hicken directed that physicians should disclose information that a reasonable person in that position would find important. In Nixdorf's case, she was not told about a surgical needle left during her operation in 1964, and this information was not disclosed until 1976 by a different provider.[19]

Most providers believe that they understand the concept of consent, but most find them extremely difficult to define. Informed consent is a fundamental and basic requirement for all procedures and treatments. It implies understanding and discussion of the nature of a given illness; the workup and therapy; risks and benefits; alternative treatments; and the option of refusing care with associated risks and benefits. The importance of informed consent is unquestioned in both legal and ethical importance; however, controversies prevail over the specifics.

To successfully achieve informed consent requires effective communication and a physician's respect for patients' autonomy when a patient is deemed to have "decision-making capacity." In addition, informed consent includes both ethical and legal requirements. Patients have the right to receive information and ask questions so that they can make decisions about their care.

USING SHARED DECISION-MAKING

Shared decision-making (SDM) is a patient-centered approach that created a paradigm shift in health care delivery. SDM is a distinct process, and while not specifically mandated, it is now frequently included when obtaining informed consent. It can be viewed as "discussion with" instead of a "disclosure to." While SDM can reduce net liability risks by improving overall communication satisfaction, it has the potential to increase provider's liability risks in certain situations described as follows[20]:

1. If there is inappropriate patient selection. For example, patients with cognitive declines, overwhelming systemic infection, and grossly distracting symptoms.
2. When employing SDM results in the departure of "standard of care" from well-accepted medical practices. Bad outcomes in these situations could easily be attributed to negligence by the physician.

Overall, the ED provider can protect themselves by being aware of best practices, local laws, as well as appropriately and accurately documenting the occurrence of SDM.[20]

THE "DIFFICULT PATIENT"

This term by itself is vague and often describes a unified category that comprises a wide variety of patients such as the violent patient, one who is a regular in the ED, a patient with a psychiatric condition (especially those who present with self-harm), the noncompliant patient, and the patient who either comes from prison or is in police custody. Self-awareness and understanding your own personal biases are crucial to treating these types of patients with the respect that they deserve. It may be an internal or external expression that increases the risk for poor medical care. Some of these external expressions also include how we misidentify these patients. For example, stigmatizing terminology, such as "a frequent flyer," can inhibit good judgment.

TIPS FOR THE INTOXICATED PATIENT

Approximately 1% of ED patients with presumed uncomplicated alcohol intoxication require critical care resources.[21]

1. If there is reasonable concern that the intoxicated patient has serious illness or lacks current capacity, do not let them leave.
2. Keep a drug or alcohol-intoxicated patient in the ED until you believe it is safe for them to leave.
   - Use Bitterman's "When in Doubt Rule," if needed. This rule is to do what you believe is right. Place the patient's best interest first and worry about the legality later.[22]
3. You cannot keep an intoxicated patient who has capacity against their will.
   - In the case of Kowalski v St. Francis Hospital and Health Centers, Mr Kowalski was brought in by a friend to the emergency department intoxicated and seeking admission to its affiliated detox facility. After waiting for transport to the detox unit, the patient told a nurse that he was going to go home. The nurse went to inform the physician and upon the return, the patient had left. Hospital security was notified. Mr Kowalski ultimately was struck by a vehicle leaving him paralyzed. He sued the hospital for malpractice and negligence as they did not keep him until his intoxication wore off. Ultimately, the court ruled that keeping an intoxicated patient against their will is false imprisonment.[23]
4. Consider and treat for reversible causes of violent behavior (eg, hypoglycemia, head injury, and intoxication).
5. The "legal ethanol limit" for driving does not indicate mental status or adequate capacity.
6. Alcohol levels may be problematic; some inexperienced drinkers may be clinically intoxicated at a blood alcohol level (BAL) of 60 g/dL while a chronic alcoholic might be in withdrawal at levels less than 250 mg/dL.
7. Sobriety is not based on a BAL, but on clinical assessment. You can use scoring systems such as Hack's impairment index to objectively track and monitor symptoms of alcohol-induced impairment. https://www.mdcalc.com/calc/10415/hacks-impairment-index-hii
8. Document your specific observations that led you to determine capacity or lack of capacity; drinking alcohol does not mean there is a lack of capacity

DOES OPIOID USE IMPAIR INFORMED CONSENT?

In acute pain secondary to surgical pathology, it is not an uncommon practice to withhold opioids until evaluated by a surgeon. However, there are no studies to date that suggest that consent obtained under the influence of opioids is invalid. In fact, withholding pain medication until the patient signs procedural consent is likely to be considered coercion. Pain medications should never be withheld from a patient to obtain informed consent. In certain situations, pain control can relieve both the physical and emotional distress allowing them to better focus on the informed consent process. However, if the pain medications cause the patient to be unable to understand, listen to, or to communicate a decision, informed consent cannot be achieved.[24]

EMERGENCY MEDICAL TREATMENT AND LABOR ACT

"Anyone," "anything," and "anytime" make emergency departments unique in medicine. However, the "anyone" became blurred. The widespread practice of "patient dumping" was a significant problem before legislation in the mid-1980s. "Patient dumping" occurs where hospitals fail to screen, treat, or appropriately transfer patients based on the uninsured patient's inability to pay for care. In the 1980s, about 250,000 people were transferred yearly based on their lack of ability to pay. Most of these patients came from private community hospitals and were transferred to public-supported county hospitals.[25] Research from Cook County Hospital in Chicago provided significant insight into the extent of patient dumping concluding that these transfers occurred for economic reasons. The main reason for initiating transfer was lack of adequate insurance in 87% of cases. Furthermore, 89% of the 467 patients transferred to Cook County Hospital were minorities and 81% were unemployed.[26] These financially motivated transfers often jeopardized patients' health due to failure to stabilize patients prior to transport and inadequate communication.

To address such issue, the United States Congressional Act passed Emergency Medical Treatment and Labor Act (EMTALA) in April 1986, as part of the Consolidated Omnibus Budget Reconciliation Act (COBRA). According to Section 9121 of COBRA, any individual who comes to the emergency department for examination or treatment, must receive a medical screening examination (MSE) within the capabilities of that hospital's department, to determine whether or not an emergency medical condition (EMC) exists. Furthermore, if there is a medical emergency, the hospital must stabilize the condition or provide appropriate transfer. The hospital is obligated to provide these services regardless of the patient's insurance status or ability to pay.[27] This applies to the physical space of the emergency department, the hospital's property, and within 250 yards of the hospital. If a patient presents for care at a clinic that is about 2 football fields away from the ED, then the staff needs to know what an MSE entails and how to properly transfer the patient to the ED for higher level care.

DEFINITIONS MATTER WHEN DEALING WITH EMERGENCY MEDICAL TREATMENT AND LABOR ACT

The term "emergency medical condition (EMC)" is defined by EMTALA as "a medical condition with acute symptoms of sufficient severity (including severe pain, psychiatric disturbances and/or symptoms of substance abuse) such that the absence of immediate medical attention could place the health of a person in serious jeopardy, serious impairment to bodily functions, or serious dysfunction to any bodily organ or part."[28]

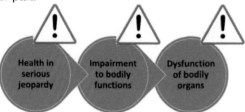

For a pregnant woman having contractions, this also means situations where there is inadequate time to effect a safe transfer to another hospital before delivery or that the transfer may pose a threat to the health or safety of the woman or the unborn child.[28] Stabilizing a patient means providing medical treatments to reasonably assure no clinical deterioration of a medical condition occurs during transfer. For a pregnant person with contractions, "stabilization" may refer to the delivery of the fetus and the placenta.[29]

Under EMTALA law, if transfer is required, it must be "appropriate." This includes

- The patient received adequate stabilization to minimize risk during transfer
- Receiving hospital accepts the transfer of the patient
- Receiving hospital must have the necessary resources and personnel
- The transferring hospital sends the receiving facility the medical records and diagnostic findings related to the emergency condition
- Must be transported with qualified personnel and equipment
- If unstable, then the physician or "qualified medical person" certifies that the benefit of transfer outweighs the risks
- If an individual is acting on their behalf and requesting transfer, then they must be aware of the risk and benefits associated with transfer[29]

WHO CAN PERFORM MEDICAL SCREENING EXAMINATIONS?

It is a common misconception that only emergency medicine physicians can perform MSEs. The short answer provided by EMTALA law is "qualified medical personnel" can provide MSEs. It is the individual hospital's governing body that decides who is authorized (some permit nurses to perform the MSE). It is important to be aware of who can perform this examination at your institution.

PARENTAL CONSENT FOR A PEDIATRIC MEDICAL SCREENING EXAMINATION

The American Academy of Pediatrics supports that all pediatrics patients should receive an initial evaluation regardless of the presence of a legally authorized decision-maker.[30] A medical screening examination or any medical care necessary to prevent significant harm to a pediatric patient should not be withheld or delayed due to issues obtaining consent.

THE "VIP" PATIENT

There are times when a private patient comes to the ED to be seen by their specialist. For example, patient X with a history of liver disease was told by his hepatologist to come to the ED and have the ED notify him to come to the ED. The patient in triage states, "I am here to see my hepatologist." This private patient, regardless of "VIP" status, should follow the same intake procedure as everyone else and needs to be triaged and processed in the same manner (this includes an MSE). The triage examination alone does not satisfy EMTALA. Once a medical screening examination determines there is no EMC, then EMTALA is satisfied, and the patient can legally await their private physician.

PREAUTHORIZATION CALLS

Patient X arrives with chest pain and abdominal pain but is worried that their insurance company will not cover their ED visit. To be helpful, the triage nurse calls their insurance company for approval.

Although insurance companies or managed care organizations are becoming more aggressive in denying payments, they cannot prevent an EM provider from performing a federally mandated MSE and stabilizing the patient. In fact, Centers for Medicare and Medicaid services (CMS) states that it is inappropriate for a hospital to request prior authorization before the MSE is completed.[31]

MODE OF TRANSFER TO ANOTHER FACILITY

EMTALA does not dictate in what mode a patient must be transferred. If it is safe for the patient to use their personal vehicles, allow them to do so. For instance, patients given opioids for pain control may not be safe to drive themselves to another facility. Those with IVs are generally transported by ambulance.

IS SEVERE PAIN CONSIDERED AN EMERGENCY MEDICAL CONDITION?

The short answer is that severe pain is not an EMC under EMTALA. The long answer is that it can be more complex. Pain is certainly a medical condition and anyone presenting with any type of pain must be medically screened. Following the definition of what constitutes an EMC (described in the earlier section), "severe pain" alone is not sufficient to be considered an EMC.[28] However, if pain could reasonably be expected to place the patient in serious jeopardy, serious impairment to bodily functions, or serious dysfunction of any organ or part, then it is classified as an EMC. If no EMC is identified, EMTALA no longer applies. There is no mandate to provide pain treatment, pain relief, or legal requirement to administer opioids under any scenario.

UNDER EMERGENCY MEDICAL TREATMENT AND LABOR ACT, IS THERE A LEGAL OBLIGATION TO REFILL PAIN MEDICATION PRESCRIPTIONS?

No. However, these patients still must undergo an MSE. If there is no EMC, then it is up to the physician's judgment to provide the refill or not.

A PATIENT HAS COME TO THE EMERGENCY DEPARTMENT ALMOST EVERY OTHER DAY FOR EVALUATION. DURING TRIAGE, CAN THAT PATIENT BE TOLD THAT THEY HAVE X NUMBER OF ED VISITS THIS YEAR?

No! Even those patients that are present regularly at the ED can experience a life-threatening event. Only after the MSE has been completed and reveals that there is no EMC, can this type of information be given to a patient. Hospitals are not allowed to "unduly discourage" a patient from receiving an MSE.

DOES EMERGENCY MEDICAL TREATMENT AND LABOR ACT APPLY TO INPATIENTS?

EMTALA continues to apply to those "admitted" to the ED, labor and delivery unit, or placed under "observation" status until they are stabilized or formally admitted to the hospital. Once they are formally admitted (and no longer in observation status), EMTALA no longer applies. CMS also considered that patients may be formally admitted yet later discharged or transferred for financial reasons or as a ruse to avoid EMTALA. To avoid these scenarios, CMS imposed a qualifying factor that admissions should be made in "good faith."[32]

DOES EMERGENCY MEDICAL TREATMENT AND LABOR ACT APPLY TO CONSULTANTS?

EMTALA is not solely for ED physicians. EMTALA citations have been made because on-call provider either failed to appear or appeared late. Although this time is not a rule according to CMS, there are states that have mandated laws that an ED specialty consultation should be within 30 minutes of being called such as in New Jersey and West Virginia.[33] This will vary in your institution so ask your hospital administration and be familiar with these expectations.

If a consultant refuses to evaluate the patient, notify them that this is an EMTALA violation as they may not be aware. In such situations, speaking to the consultant on a recorded line, documenting both the discussion and all efforts made to obtain on-call consultation are helpful. The ED physician should not be subject to sanctions if an unstable patient had to be transferred because the on-call provider did not respond.[33]

EMERGENCY MEDICAL TREATMENT AND LABOR ACT AND PATIENTS LEAVING AGAINST MEDICAL ADVICE

There are no clear guidelines or EMTALA regulations for patients leaving AMA. There is no EMTALA violation if leaving AMA as long as the patient with capacity does so of their own free will without coercion. A patient who has capacity can also refuse to consent to treatment and/or transfer. A hospital is deemed to meet their requirements if they properly offered treatment, informed the individual of the risks and benefits, and took all reasonable steps to secure informed consent refusal.[27]

HOW IS EMERGENCY MEDICAL TREATMENT AND LABOR ACT ENFORCED?

Enforcement of this "antidumping" law is done by civil money penalties and civil enforcement. Enforcement is through the CMS and the Office of the Inspector General (OIG) of the Department of Health and Human Services. The process begins when a Certified Medical Examiner receives a complaint from any source. If CMS agrees to investigate, then a state survey agency will visit the hospital unannounced. CMS can then initiate a 90 day termination process (or 23 day if there is an immediate or serious threat). Hospitals have this period to submit a plan of correction, and if accepted, it can end the termination process. Once the termination process has occurred, CMS forwards the case to the OIG for possible civil monetary penalties.

There are 3 classes of penalties when violating EMTALA: monetary, exclusion, and civil suit. The subject of a monetary penalty can be to the participating hospital and/or the physician involved. Per violation, a penalty can be received on a hospital of US$119,942 for hospitals over 100 beds and US$59,973 for hospitals under 100 beds. For physicians, a penalty of US$119,942 per violation can be received.[27] Currently, there is a 2 year statute of limitations for civil enforcement of any violation.[34] This fine is not covered by malpractice insurance. Penalties can also exclude the hospital or physician from participation in Medicare and State health care programs. Finally, private citizens harmed by this can file a civil suit under the personal injury laws of that state in which the hospital is located.[27]

Penalties against individual physicians are rare. In an analysis of all civil monetary penalty settlements between 2002 and 2015 relating to EMTALA violations, only 4% were cited against individual physicians while 96% against facilities. Of those penalties against individual physicians, most involved the on-call specialist including obstetricians and surgical specialist rather than emergency physicians.[35]

HOW DOES ONE REPORT A VIOLATION?

Any individual can report a suspected EMTALA violation, and a report can be filed anonymously. This can be done by reaching out to the local Centers for Medicare & Medicaid Services State Survey Agency to let them know you would like to file an EMTALA complaint. There are 10 Regional offices across the United States with each covering certain states.

AN EXAMPLE OF EMERGENCY MEDICAL TREATMENT AND LABOR ACT VIOLATION

In 2018, an Alabama hospital entered into a US$80,000 settlement after failure to adequately screen for an emergency medicine condition and provide the necessary stabilizing treatment. The patient had requested to see a physician and became belligerent when staff asked further questions leading to being escorted out of the emergency department. Upon return, the patient's girlfriend drove to the ambulance bay stating that the patient had a seizure and was informed by staff that they had to leave. The patient's girlfriend drove him to a subsequent hospital but was pronounced dead shortly after arrival.

WHEN IS MEDICAL SCREENING EXAMINATION NOT REQUIRED?

If a person presents to the ED requesting preventive care services or brought in under police custody with request for gathering of evidence for criminal law cases, then the hospital is not obligated to provide an MSE. Examples include immunizations, rabies vaccine series, allergy shots, flu shots, and blood alcohol tests.

Attention to detail is instrumental when determining if an MSE is needed. For example, if an individual was involved in a motor vehicle accident and the chief complaint is "here for just a blood alcohol test" this scenario warrants an MSE to determine if an EMC exists. One should also consider that the patient that appears intoxicated may be hypoglycemic, have a head injury, or have other medical causes of being altered. Another example is the patient following up for a rabies vaccine series as they may have a wound infection. So, despite the narrow exclusion for MSE, the safer option for the ED provider is to always perform an MSE regardless of reason.

CLINICS CARE POINTS

- Perform a timely MSE in all patients.
- Say "No" to the preauthorization approval process. But if done, it *must* be after the MSE.
- Parental consent is not a prerequisite for a pediatric MSE.
- Diagnosing an EMC is not enough; patients must be stabilized to the best of the ability of the resources of the ED/hospital.
- Admissions should be in good faith.
- EMTALA continues in those admitted to the ED, labor and delivery, and those in "observation".
- Anyone can file an EMTALA complaint.
- After stabilizing the EMC to the best of the hospital's capability, you can transfer unstable patients to a higher level of care if the benefits outweigh the risks.
- Hospitals with specialized services are required to accept transfers if they have the capacity to do so.
- Be aware of who can provide an MSE at your institution.
- Assume you are always responsible for the patient.
- Always err on the side of what is best for the patient.

DISCLOSURE

The authors have nothing to disclose.

REFERENCES

1. Hodgins MJ, Moore N, Little J. Those who opt to leave: Comparison by triage acuity of emergency patients who leave prior to seeing a medical practitioner. International Emergency Nursing 2023;70:101349.
2. Li DR, Brennan JJ, Kreshak AA, et al. Patients who leave the emergency department without being seen and their follow-up behavior: a retrospective descriptive analysis. J Emerg Med 2019;57(1):106–13.
3. Sheraton M, Gooch C, Kashyap R. Patients leaving without being seen from the emergency department: a prediction model using machine learning on a nationwide database. J Am Coll Emerg Physicians Open 2020;1(6):1684–90.
4. Hsia RY, Asch SM, Weiss RE, et al. Hospital determinants of emergency department left without being seen Rates. Ann Emerg Med 2011;58(1):24–32, e3.
5. National Center for Health Statistics. NCHS Fact Sheet June 2019. 2019. Available at: https://www.cdc.gov/nchs/data/factsheets/factsheet_nhcs.pdf.
6. Cairns C, Kang K. National Center for Health Statistics. National Hospital Ambulatory Medical Care Survey: 2021 Emergency Department Summary Tables. Available at: https://www.cdc.gov/nchs/data/nhamcs/web_tables/2021-nhamcs-ed-web-tables-508.pdf.
7. Janke AT, Melnick ER, Venkatesh AK. Monthly Rates of Patients Who Left Before Accessing Care in US Emergency Departments, 2017-2021. JAMA Netw Open 2022;5(9):e2233708. https://doi.org/10.1001/jamanetworkopen.2022.33708.
8. Sember M, Donley C, Eggleston M. Implementation of a provider in triage and its effect on left without being seen rate at a community trauma center. Open Access Emerg Med 2021;13:137–41.
9. Hsieh A, Arena A, Oraha A, et al. Implementation of vertical split flow model for patient throughput at a community hospital emergency department. J Emerg Med 2023;64(1):77–82.
10. Scolnik D, Matthews P, Caulfeild J, et al. Pagers in a busy paediatric emergency waiting room: A randomized controlled trial. Paediatr Child Health 2003;8(7):422–6.
11. Smalley CM, Meldon SW, Simon EL, et al. Emergency department patients who leave before treatment is complete. West J Emerg Med 2021;22(2):148–55. https://doi.org/10.5811/westjem.2020.11.48427.
12. Ali S, Colucciello S. Informed Consent/Against Medical Advice (AMA). In: Johnson W, Nordt S, Mattu A, et al, editors. CorePendium. Burbank, CA: CorePendium, LLC; 2023. Available at: https://www.emrap.org/corependium/chapter/rec5lasj250M4e58d/Informed-ConsentAgainst-Medical-Advice-AMA. [Accessed 11 April 2024].
13. Choi M, Kim H, Qian H, et al, Readmission rates of patients discharged against medical advice: a matched cohort study. PLoS One 2011;6(9):e24459. https://doi.org/10.1371/journal.pone.0024459.
14. Tsai J, Janke AT, Krumholz HM, et al. Race and ethnicity and emergency department discharge against medical advice. JAMA Netw Open 2023;6(11):e2345437.
15. Schaefer GR, Matus H, Schumann JH, et al. Financial responsibility of hospitalized patients who left against medical advice: medical urban legend? J Gen Intern Med 2012;27(7):825–30. https://doi.org/10.1007/s11606-012-1984-x.
16. Bazzano LA, Durant J, Brantley PR. A Modern History of Informed Consent and the Role of Key Information. Ochsner J 2021;21(1):81–5. https://doi.org/10.31486/toj.19.0105.

17. Classic case articulating the reasonable patient standard - Canterbury v. Spence., 464 F.2d 772 (D.C. Cir. 1972). Available at: https://biotech.law.lsu.edu/cases/consent/canterbury_v_spence.htm.
18. Moore GP, Matlock AG, Kiley JL, et al. Emergency Physicians: Beware of the Consent Standard of Care. Clin Pract Cases Emerg Med 2018;2(2):109–11.
19. Brief of Appellant, Nixdorf v. Hicken, No. 16151 (Utah Supreme Court, 1979).
20. Lindor RA, Kunneman M, Hanzel M, et al. Consent in the Context of Shared Decision Making. Acad Emerg Med 2016;23(12):1428–33.
21. Klein LR, Cole JB, Driver BE, et al. Unsuspected Critical Illness Among Emergency Department Patients Presenting for Acute Alcohol Intoxication. Ann Emerg Med 2018;71(3):279–88.
22. Bitterman R. Against Medical Advice. Epix Principles. November 2011.
23. Kowalski v St. Francis Hosp. & Health Ctrs. (2013 NY Slip Op 04756). Available at: https://www.nycourts.gov/REPORTER/3dseries/2013/2013_04756.htm.
24. Lucha PA Jr, Kropcho L, Schneider JJ, et al. Acute pain and narcotic use does not impair the ability to provide informed consent: evaluation of a competency assessment tool in the acute pain patient. Am Surg 2006;72(2):154–7.
25. The EMTALA story. Available at: https://www.emra.org/books/advocacy-handbook/emtala-story.
26. Schiff RL, Ansell DA, Schlosser JE, et al. Transfers to a public hospital. A prospective study of 467 patients. N Engl J Med 1986;314(9):552–7. https://doi.org/10.1056/NEJM198602273140905.
27. Understanding EMTALA. ACEP.org. Available at: https://www.acep.org/life-as-a-physician/ethics–legal/emtala/emtala-fact-sheet.
28. Directors, Quality, Safety & Oversight Group (QSOG) and Survey & Operations Group (SOG). Reinforcement of EMTALA Obligations Specific to Patients Who Are Pregnant or Are Experiencing Pregnancy Loss. 2022. Available at: https://www.cms.gov/files/document/qso-22-22-hospitals.pdf.
29. Lulla A, Svancarek B. EMS USA Emergency Medical Treatment and Active Labor Act. StatPearls - NCBI Bookshelf. 2022. Available at: https://www.ncbi.nlm.nih.gov/books/NBK539798/.
30. Katz AL, Webb SA. Informed Consent in Decision-Making in Pediatric practice. Pediatrics 2016;138(2).
31. Centers for Medicare & Medicaid Services. State Operations Manual Appendix V – Interpretive Guidelines – Responsibilities of Medicare Participating Hospitals in Emergency Cases. 2019. Available at: https://www.cms.gov/regulations-and-guidance/guidance/manuals/downloads/som107ap_v_emerg.pdf.
32. Bitterman R. Does EMTALA really end when a hospital admits an ED patient?
33. Zibulewsky J. The Emergency Medical Treatment and Active Labor Act (EMTALA): what it is and what it means for physicians. SAVE Proc 2001;14(4):339–46. https://doi.org/10.1080/08998280.2001.11927785.
34. Impact of EMTALA. Available at: https://www.emra.org/books/advocacy-handbook-2019/impact-of-emtala.
35. Terp S, Wang B, Raffetto B, et al. Individual Physician Penalties Resulting From Violation of Emergency Medical Treatment and Labor Act: A Review of Office of the Inspector General Patient Dumping Settlements, 2002-2015. Acad Emerg Med 2017;24(4):442–6. https://doi.org/10.1111/acem.13159.

Clinical Practice Guidelines and Medical Malpractice Risk

Christopher E. San Miguel, MD, MEd*

KEYWORDS

- Clinical practice guidelines • Medical malpractice • Malpractice defense
- Malpractice claim • Litigation

KEY POINTS

- When admissible as evidence, clinical practice guidelines (CPGs) are used as both inculpatory and exculpatory evidence, though much more commonly as the former.
- Providing care compliant with a CPG does not grant the clinician immunity from tortious litigation, but it can deter plaintiff's attorneys from taking the case and provide the foundation for a strong legal defense.
- There are several potential arguments that can be made to justify the deviation from the CPG. Effective communication with patients and strong, comprehensive documentation help to defend care that is noncompliant with a CPG.

INTRODUCTION

The Clinical Case

A 75-year-old gentleman is brought to the emergency department (ED) by ambulance with a concern for a stroke. Thirty minutes prior to arrival, the patient was standing in line at the grocery store when he suddenly fell to the ground. The paramedics noted a facial droop, right sided weakness, and difficulty speaking, so they initiated a field activated stroke alert. On arrival, the Emergency Physician (EP) confirms the neurologic deficits and calculates a National Institutes of Health (NIH) Stroke Scale score of 17. His glucose is 105, and his head computed tomography (CT) does not show any significant abnormalities. The patient has a full medical record available for review, and he does not seem to have any contraindication to lytic therapy. The EP attempts to contact family but is unsuccessful. The patient has significant receptive and productive aphasia and is unable to consent for treatment. The institution's clinical practice guideline (CPG) for ischemic stroke states, "In cases of severe neurologic deficits, which result in a loss of medical decision-making capacity, the treating provider may consider administering

Department of Emergency Medicine, The Ohio State University College of Medicine
* 783 Prior Hall, 376 W 10th Ave, Columbus, OH, 43210
E-mail address: Christopher.sanmiguel@osumc.edu

Emerg Med Clin N Am 43 (2025) 155–161
https://doi.org/10.1016/j.emc.2024.05.029   emed.theclinics.com
0733-8627/25/© 2024 Elsevier Inc. All rights are reserved, including those for text and data mining, AI training, and similar technologies.

lytic therapy under emergent implied consent if no surrogate decision maker for the patient can be promptly found." After careful consideration, the EP orders the lytic therapy and prepares the patient for transport to a comprehensive stroke center. Unfortunately, the patient's neurologic status worsens en route, and on arrival to the stroke center he is found to have a large intraparenchymal hemorrhage. Despite resuscitative efforts, the patient passes away a few hours later. Several months later, the patient's wife contacts an attorney to explore a possible medical malpractice suit against the EP.

Is the EP insulated from lawsuits because his care was in accordance with the CPG? What if the EP's care had deviated from the CPG? Would this result in increased liability exposure?

BACKGROUND

CPGs have become increasingly popular to promote patient safety and to help clinicians provide evidence-based care to their patients.[1] The Institute of Medicine defines CPGs as "statements that include recommendations, intended to optimize patient care, that are informed by a systematic review of evidence and an assessment of the benefits and harms of alternative care options."[2] CPGs can be created at the department or institution level, but national and international professional organizations such as the American Heart Association and the American College of Emergency Physicians also create and publish CPGs.

While CPGs were never meant to replace individual clinical judgment, deviation from them is often examined when there is a negative patient outcome.[3] Indeed, this problem was foreseen when such guidelines were first popularized in the 1990s.[3] The medical establishment expressed significant concern that these guidelines would be used punitively against physicians whose practice varied from the published document, whether that variation was justified or not. In fact, to promote development of CPGs and garner support from physicians, some state legislatures developed programs which granted physicians immunity from medical malpractice claims as long as the care provided was consistent with a CPG; these programs have all since been retired, and interestingly were rarely utilized.[3]

Medical Malpractice Litigation

The appeal of using a CPG as evidence in a medical malpractice case is that it provides an unbiased, evidence-based benchmark against which the care in question can be measured. This speaks to 1 of the 4 main elements of a medical malpractice case, the breach of duty. In order to be successful in their lawsuit, the plaintiff must demonstrate that the physician did not provide the standard of care in fulfilling their duty to treat the patient in a competent manner.[4] Exactly how the standard of care is defined varies from jurisdiction to jurisdiction, but in general, it refers to the care which a similarly trained physician in a similar circumstance would have reasonably provided.[2] The breach of duty can be difficult to impossible to definitively prove as both sides in the lawsuit will hire one or more experts who will testify the care provided did (from the defendant side) or did not (from the plaintiff's side) meet the standard of care. Particularly to a lay jury, contradicting experts support the defendant's default argument that the care provided was a reasonable option and therefore followed the standard of care. In contrast to dueling experts, the CPG provides a single consensus opinion on how best to care for a specific patient population or pathology. Even when instructed to the contrary, it is easy to see how a jury may assign undue weight to whether the physician followed a CPG in providing the care in question.

But before considering how CPGs are utilized in malpractice suits, it needs to be determined whether CPGs can even *be* utilized in malpractice suits. Because CPGs are considered out-of-court statements, they are considered hearsay evidence.[2] In general, hearsay evidence is not admissible in court. However, numerous exclusions and exceptions exist, and like much of United States law, they vary by jurisdiction. The rules and regulations surrounding hearsay evidence are complicated, nuanced, and frankly beyond the scope of this discussion. Suffice to say that depending on the jurisdiction and how the CPG is being introduced as evidence it may or may not be admissible.[2] Furthermore, the amount of evidentiary weight granted to a CPG varies from jurisdiction to jurisdiction. In most of the country, a CPG (if admissible) can be considered along with other evidence, such as expert testimony, to collectively define the standard of care. Rarely, is it automatically considered to establish the standard of care once entered into evidence.[1] In circumstances where the CPG is not permitted into evidence, it becomes a moot point whether the care that was provided was consistent or not, as the jury will be unaware of the CPG's existence.

The general trend in courtrooms has been to increasingly allow CPGs to be entered into evidence and juries to consider them in making their determinations.[1] Plaintiff's attorneys attempt to use CPGs as inculpatory evidence to demonstrate deviation from the standard of care.[5] For instance, in our clinical example, if the institution's CPG stated that "either the patient or their surrogate decision maker must consent to lytic therapy," the plaintiff's attorneys would likely argue that the physician should be held liable for the patient's poor outcome because he failed to follow the standard of care, as evidence by his failure to obtain consent as recommended in the CPG. In contrast, defense attorneys attempt to use CPGs as exculpatory evidence to demonstrate that the physician provided the standard of care.[5] In our case, the physician's attorneys would likely argue that the physician should not be held liable for the patient's poor outcome because he followed the standard of care, as evidenced by providing care under implied emergent consent when no surrogate decision maker was promptly available, as directed by the CPG.

DISCUSSION
Academic Study of Clinical Practice Guidelines and Medical Malpractice

In 1995, Hyams and colleagues sought to determine how CPGs are most often utilized in malpractice cases.[6] The researchers examined 259 claims opened against physicians involving 2 malpractice insurance carriers between 1990 and 1992. All the cases were reviewed for the use of CPGs as evidence. Of the 259 cases, 17 involved CPGs. In 12 cases, the use of the CPG was in an inculpatory fashion (implying guilt), compared to 4 cases in which the CPG was used in as exculpatory evidence (relieving of guilt).[6] The use of the CPG in 1 case was classified as indeterminate. Of the 12 inculpatory cases, 1 case went to trial and the jury returned a verdict for the defendant, 8 cases were settled with payment to the plaintiff, 1 case was closed with no payment, and 2 cases remained open at the time of the research. Of the 4 exculpatory cases, 1 case went to trial and the jury returned a verdict for the plaintiff, 1 case was settled with payment to the plaintiff, and 2 cases remained open at the time of the research.[6] In addition to reviewing malpractice cases, these researchers also distributed a survey to medical malpractice attorneys about their experiences with CPGs. Defense attorneys answered that of their cases which involved CPG, 54% of cases involved deviation from the CPG, 23% of cases exhibited care which complied with a CPG, and in 23% of cases adherence to the CPG was disputed.[6] The researchers concluded that CPGs are used as both inculpatory and exculpatory evidence, but it is far more common for them to be used as inculpatory evidence.[6]

These findings were supported in a subsequent study by 3 of the same researchers.[5] Searching a national database of US court cases from 1980 to 1994, the researchers reviewed any case which mentioned any of the 54 professional societies and government agencies that were known to issue CPGs at that time.[5] They found a total of 37 cases involving CPGs. In 29 cases, the use of the CPG was inculpatory, compared to 8 cases in which the use of the CPG was exculpatory.[5]

From a broad perspective, this disproportionate use of CPGs as inculpatory evidence makes sense. It stands to reason, that following a CPG is at least the beginnings of a strong potential defense. We can therefore expect that at least some potential cases in which the physician follows the CPG (and the CPG would presumably be used as exculpatory evidence), do not progress to the point that they are included in insurance or court databases. Indeed, as part of the Hyam and colleagues survey, plaintiff's attorneys were asked about whether CPG compliance influenced their decision to take medical malpractice case. Just over a quarter of plaintiff's attorneys, reported that in the past year a CPG had influenced their decision not to take a case at least once.[6] Similarly, just over 30% of the plaintiff's attorneys reported that in the past year a CPG had influenced their decision to bring at least 1 case.[6]

Ransom and colleagues attempted to expand upon the work of Hyam by completing a case control study of obstetrics-related malpractice cases.[7] They examined 290 malpractice claims and 262 control delivery cases from a single health system from 1988 to 1998. They found that the care provided in the malpractice complaints did not comply with the institutional CPG in 43% of cases.[7] In contrast only 12% of the control cases did not comply the institutional CPG.[7] They concluded that adherence to CPG might reduce malpractice exposure for both the individual physician and the institution. Of note, the conclusion is weakened by the fact that the institutional CPG was not implemented until the last year of the study period. While the cases prior to this were measured against the CPG by the researchers, adherence to the CPG did not actual influence any of the legal cases as the CPG did not yet exist. It would be most accurate to say that this work demonstrated that lower-quality clinical care (as defined by its eventual noncompliance with a CPG) was more often found in malpractice cases than in control cases.

In summary, several reviews of malpractice cases and a survey of malpractice attorneys have demonstrated.

1. Compliance (and noncompliance) with CPG has an impact on plaintiff's attorney's decision to pursue a case.
2. CPGs are used in both inculpatory and exculpatory evidence, but much more commonly as the former.
3. Clinical care that was, in retrospect, noncompliant with a CPG was found more often in malpractice cases than control cases.

Legal Defense Strategies

As discussed above, in only rare circumstances are CPGs given sufficient evidentiary weight to allow a malpractice case to be determined solely based on whether the care in question was compliant or not.[1] It stands to reason then there are several potential defense arguments that can be made to justify the deviation of the clinical care provided. While it is unimportant for the EP to understand the details of forming a legal strategy, it is helpful to understand how real time documentation of the clinical care can impact a potential subsequent malpractice lawsuit.

Although there are no academic papers published specifically examining the role of documentation in CPG noncompliance and its effect on malpractice litigation, it is a universally held belief that the more of the original thought process and clinical decision making that is documented, the stronger the potential defense will be.[4] To this end, it is recommended that physicians take the time to thoroughly document their clinical decision making and explicitly state why they are deviating from a CPG within the patient's medical record. At the very least, this demonstrates the physician's knowledge of the CPG and that they attempted to provide thoughtful, individualized medical care for the patient. It also serves to undercut potential, plaintiff's attorney's narratives that the physician was unaware of a CPG which they should have known about or that the physician simply ignored the CPG in caring for the patient.

One of the main arguments presented in cases of CPG noncompliance challenges the underlying assumption that the CPG represents the standard of care. The legal definition of the standard of care varies by jurisdiction, but most often is reduced to reasonable and ordinary care that a physician of similar training in a similar circumstance would customarily provide. It has been argued (successfully, at times) that CPGs represent ideal or aspirational care which far exceeds the standard of care.[1] Therefore, it is quite possible for a physician to provide the standard of care while also not following the CPG.[8] Admittedly, this particular defense would be difficult to document in the medical record and the physician would want to avoid documenting anything to the effect of "I know that I could be providing better, aspirational care, but I have chosen not to." However, if there are circumstances outside of the physician's control which are influencing the level or quality of care that can be provided, this along with the physician's attempt to change the circumstances should be documented.

For instance, a rural hospital has a CPG that states all acute stroke patients should be transferred within 90 minutes of arrival to the ED. Immediately after seeing the patient and ordering thrombolytic therapy, the EP arranges for air transport to the closest stroke center. Unfortunately, as the helicopter touches down at the rural hospital, it has engine trouble and is unable to safely transport the patient. Strictly speaking, the patient's care will be noncompliant with the CPG as the transfer is delayed. In this circumstance, the EP should document the time that the original transport was arranged, the time that they became aware that the original transport was not available, and subsequent attempts to transfer the patient as quickly as possible.

Another commonly deployed defense is to argue that the care provided was more individualized than the CPG. It is impossible for a CPG to account for every possible patient, pathology, or facility factor which could influence the provided clinical care.[8] In fact, it is helpful that CPGs themselves often contain verbiage attesting to this very limitation. Documentation is very helpful when making this argument. Imagine an EP is treating a patient for otitis externa. The CPG may recommend Antibiotic A, but the patient is uninsured and tells the EP that they will be unable to afford this medication. Antibiotic B is less efficacious than Antibiotic A, but much more affordable. Reasoning that the patient is unlikely to receive any of Antibiotic A if prescribed, the EP prescribes Antibiotic B. This reasoning along with the conversation with the patient discussing the treatment options should be thoroughly documented.

A similar, successful defense argument is that the medical care described in the CPG does not represent the only acceptable course of action. This is called a respectable minority defense.[4] In this defense, it is accepted that the CPG represents a majority opinion and should be considered a standard of care. However, it argues that a respectable number of peers of the defendant would agree that another care plan is equally valid and should also be considered a standard of care.[4] Management of stable atrial fibrillation with rapid ventricular response illustrates this point well. Local custom and an institutional CPG may recommend rate control as a preferred first line therapy. However, rhythm control in the form of electrical or chemical cardioversion is another acceptable course of action. In fact, the defense attorneys may submit a national CPG, which acknowledges the validity of this treatment option to bolster the respectable minority defense. Further supporting this defense, is that surprisingly few published CPG comply with the Institute of Medicine's standards for CPG development. They often fail to report conflicts of interest, criteria for and selection process of committee members are rarely described, the committees often do not include an information scientist or patient representative, and differences of opinion between committee members are rarely reported.[9]

The assumption of risk defense argues that the physician should not be held liable for a course of treatment if the plaintiff agreed to that treatment.[4] Paramount to this defense is that the patient must fully understand the potential risks and benefits of both treatment options. It is incumbent upon the physician to discuss the risks and benefits with patients and help them make an informed decision. For instance, if a patient presents with a cellulitis, the EP may discuss treatment with oral antibiotics as an outpatient versus inpatient treatment with intravenous antibiotics, despite a CPG recommending that the patient be admitted to the hospital. Documenting this conversation and the patient's ultimate decision can shift the responsibility from the EP to the patient.[4]

BACK TO THE CASE

Back to the original case vignette; is the EP insulated from lawsuits because his care complied with the institutional CPG? Based on the current evidence, it is difficult to tease apart whether the presence of a CPG or simply providing quality care which happens to comply with a CPG is protective. However, it is clear that providing care that complies with a CPG is less likely to lead to a malpractice case. While rarely assigned enough evidentiary weight to justify a summary judgment for the physician, introducing a CPG as exculpatory evidence provides a strong foundation to argue that the defendant met the standard of care.

Does providing care outside of the CPG result in increased liability? At the claims and trial stages of malpractice cases, the most common use of a CPG is as inculpatory evidence to demonstrate that the physician did not follow the standard of care. It is a reasonable conclusion to say that not following a CPG does increase the risk of malpractice litigation. This risk, however, can be mitigated by high-quality communication with the patient and comprehensive charting of the clinical decision making during the clinical encounter.

SUMMARY

- When admissible as evidence, CPGs are used as both inculpatory and exculpatory evidence, though much more commonly as the former (ie, a higher legal risk for not following the guidelines).
- Providing care compliant with a CPG does not grant the clinician complete immunity from tortious litigation, but it can deter plaintiff's attorneys from taking the case and provide the foundation for a strong legal defense.
- There are several potential arguments that can be made to justify the deviation from the CPG, and they are rooted in effective communication and strong, comprehensive documentation.

CLINICS CARE POINTS

Medical Malpractice can be minimized by exhibiting the follow behviors:

- When it is in the patient's best interest, follow the CPG.
- When it is in the patient's best interest, don't follow the CPG.
- Thoroughly document your reasoning for deviating from the CPG.

REFERENCES

1. Mello MM. Of swords and shields: the role of clinical practice guidelines in medical malpractice litigation. Univ Penn Law Rev 2001;149(3):645–710.
2. Taylor C. The use of clinical practice guidelines in determining standard of care. J Leg Med 2014;35(2):273–90.
3. Begel J. Maine physician practice guidelines: implications for medical malpractice litigation. Maine Law Rev 1995;47:69.
4. Hudson MJ, Moore GP. Defenses to malpractice: what every emergency physician should know. J Emerg Med 2011;41(6):598–606.
5. Hyams AL, Shapiro DW, Brennan TA. Medical practice guidelines in malpractice litigation: an early retrospective. J Health Polit Policy Law 1996;21(2):289–314.
6. Hyams AL, Brandenburg JA, Lipsitz SR, et al. Practice guidelines and malpractice litigation: a two-way street. Ann Intern Med 1995;122(6):450–5.
7. Ransom SB, Studdert DM, Dombrowski MP, et al. Reduced medicolegal risk by compliance with obstetric clinical pathways: a case–control study. Obstet Gynecol 2003;101(4):751–5.
8. Vukmir RB. Policy/procedure. In: Legal issues in emergency medicine. Cambridge medicine. Cambridge University Press; 2018. Available at: https://proxy.lib.ohio-state.edu/login?url=https://search.ebscohost.com/login.aspx?direct=true&db=cat01905a&AN=ohiolink.b41021198&site=eds-live&scope=site.
9. Kung J, Miller RR, Mackowiak PA. Failure of clinical practice guidelines to meet institute of medicine standards: Two more decades of little, if any, progress. Arch Intern Med 2012;172(21):1628–33.

Reflections from a Medical Malpractice Defense Attorney

Insights on Avoiding Claims and Lawsuits

Terry Marc Calvert, JD*

KEYWORDS

- Claims • Lawsuits • Bedside manner • Legal considerations • Bottom line

KEY POINTS

- Claims and lawsuits are often triggered by dissatisfaction of patients and their families.
- Clinical judgment, record keeping, and bedside manner are key factors in whether dissatisfaction occurs and whether claims and lawsuits are pursued.
- Lawyers who agree to pursue medical lawsuits base their decisions, in part, on the contents of the medical records.
- The emergency department (ED) is unique in its activity level, pace, intensity, and the relative lack of control over which patients seek care.
- Unique aspects of the ED including acuity and volume may lead to an increase in diagnostic errors, communication issues, and dissatisfied patients, which can increase the risk for claims and lawsuits.

AVOIDING CLAIMS AND LAWSUITS
Making the Mark

As the story goes, circa 1920, Henry Ford had a big problem.[1] A gigantic generator at his auto plant would not work, and his engineers could not solve it. Ford reached out for help from Charles Steinmetz, a genius engineer who worked with Thomas Edison and General Electric. Steinmetz agreed to help and spent 2 days and nights at the plant in Michigan, evaluating the problem.

He solved it. At around 4 feet tall, he asked for a ladder and climbed up on the generator and made a chalk mark where the problem was. He told the Ford engineers what needed to be replaced under the mark, and the generator worked perfectly.

Attorney at Law, Calvert, Leever, & Ostler, 15201 Mason Road, Suite 350, Cypress, TX 77433, USA
* 20734 East Farwood Terrace, Cypress, Texas 77433.
E-mail address: marc.calvert@calvertfirm.com

Emerg Med Clin N Am 43 (2025) 163–177
https://doi.org/10.1016/j.emc.2024.05.031
0733-8627/25/© 2024 Elsevier Inc. All rights are reserved, including those for text and data mining, AI training, and similar technologies.

emed.theclinics.com

Henry Ford was thrilled! Then he got the bill from GE for US$10,000. A little surprised at the lack of detail for what was then a rather large sum, Ford balked at paying it until he received an itemized explanation for the bill.

When apprised of the request, Charles Steinmetz decided to respond personally. He took a moment to handwrite on the bill a concise, and precise, itemization of charges:

- Making the chalk mark on generator: US$1
- Knowing where to make the chalk mark: US$9999
  Henry Ford paid the bill.

Application

Having defended and helped health care providers since 1987, I believe that the bottom line in avoiding claims and lawsuits consists of knowing where to make the mark. I would offer that there are 3 key areas for making the mark in the right spot:

- Clinical judgment
- Documentation
- Bedside manner

Claims and Lawsuits

What is a "claim," and how does it relate to a "lawsuit"? A claim involves an assertion or demand. It can be as simple as a phone call expressing concerns or objections, or perhaps a written communication setting out the facts of a situation for which redress is being sought. So, in the big picture, a lawsuit is simply a more formal claim that is made in the court system.

There are many other claims besides lawsuits. A patient can send an initial letter of complaint to a physician, the physicians' group, or the institution where they work. A patient or family member may file a complaint with the licensing board in a particular state concerning the care provided by a doctor. A complaint can be made on social media. Claims can be at the core of peer review investigations, or investigations by hospitals or insurance companies regarding care complained of by patients or family.

Impact of Claims

There are many reasons for steps to be taken to avoid claims including the obvious direct professional and psychological impact. The filing of a claim against the doctor, even if it goes away on its own, arguably creates a negative mark on the record. A loss run by risk management or insurance companies will often list claims made about a provider, even if they went nowhere, and this listing may be viewed as a negative to that physician.

Further, steps typically need to be taken to defend a claim, even if it remains in-house with the hospital, group, or insurance company. This can include obtaining records, having the matter reviewed by an attorney or medical experts, and dealing with the claimant or their attorney. This process of time spent, and effort exerted, has an impact on the doctor and the doctor's record. It may manifest via a bump in insurance premium rates and may be reviewed when insurance is being renewed.

Another direct impact of a claim can include the expense related to the resolution that may be simply a reimbursement of out-of-pocket money, which the patient had to pay to cover the costs of care, but could end up being a monetary settlement with the patient to resolve the dispute including compensation for physical pain, mental anguish, and loss of earnings.

This sum is typically paid by the insurance company, but rarely rolls onto the doctor if the amount exceeds policy limits.

The Ride

The indirect impact of claims can also be more than a mere nuisance. Claims about care may cause a great deal of stress on health care providers. Claims that do not remain private can affect how a professional is viewed by others, including their peers, and by those whose opinions can affect the defendant's career, such as leadership at hospitals or by malpractice carriers. Physicians can purchase insurance coverage to cover anticipated indemnity payments, but their insurance cannot soften the indirect costs of claims such as time, stress, work, and reputational damage.[2]

It is common for there to be a significant amount of effort spent by the physician in dealing with a claim. The mantra of the police shows from the 1960s was commonly "you may beat the rap, but you are not going to beat the ride" (**Fig. 1**). This is certainly true in the arena of health care claims.

Most would agree that the process of simply going through it, the so-called ride, is unpleasant at best and a nightmare at worst. Even ultimately prevailing, such as at a jury trial or when the medical board finally dismisses the complaint, is not going to bring back the time or the worry that was lost along the way.

The legal arena can be odious for physicians whose care is being challenged. My clients are usually surprised at the acrimony and the unpredictability. One unpleasant exposure to the legal system can starkly remind one of the need to take steps to avoid a second claim.

Why are Claims Brought?

There is an array of human emotions that surface when there is an adverse outcome, but the overarching theme is dissatisfaction among patients and/or family members.[3] I see 3 repetitive reasons for such dissatisfaction leading to claims: a bad result; a savvy or litigious patient or family; and a poor bedside manner by the provider.

In my experience, at least 2 of these factors are present. If there is an adverse outcome, a litigious or sophisticated family may well pounce and utilize the system to pursue a claim or lawsuit. Even with a good bedside manner, these synergistic forces might prevail. But we cannot control the mindset of a patient or family who is litigious; we *can* control our response to traits inherent to the human condition, that is, bedside manner, a determining factor in many claims and lawsuits that are brought.[4]

The emergency room (ER) is unique terrain, with its mix of complexity, communication challenges and breakdowns, and, at times, chaos.[5] It is unusual for the health care

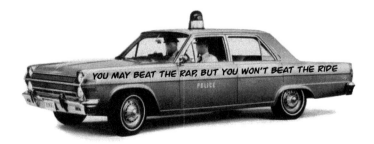

Fig. 1. Even if you beat the rap, the ride is a bumpy one.

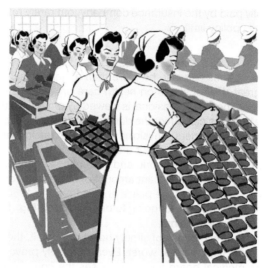

Fig. 2. Too many and too fast can lead to mistakes, and furious patients.

providers in the emergency department (ED) to have any previous connection or familiarity with the patient. This often-frenetic scene leads to an increase in the potential for mistakes. Why?

Fast can Lead to Furious

There is an episode of the famous *I Love Lucy* television series where Lucy and her friend Ethel are working at a chocolate factory (**Fig. 2**). Of course, the treadmill carrying the chocolates is too fast for them to be able to wrap them, and they soon become overwhelmed with the pace. Out of breath, Lucy remarks "Ethel, I think we are fighting a losing game."

When they hear the boss coming, they start putting chocolates in their shirts, their hats, and even eating them, to avoid failing to meet the expectations and demands. The boss comes in, seemingly satisfied that they have apparently been able to keep the pace, and yells to whoever is operating the treadmill "speed it up a little"!

It is a classic, and it is funny, and it is emblematic of our work life. In the ED, providing quality care can collide with the pressures of inadequate information and increasing demands on limited time, inhibiting our potential to make an accurate diagnosis, "error in diagnosis" being the leading cause of malpractice lawsuits.[6]

The ED can be a runaway treadmill, creating a time crunch that may impede data gathering or bedside interaction, potentially causing anger in patients and families. In addition to time/flow considerations, the patient population in the ED may demonstrate additional difficulties including intoxication, head injuries, and advanced chronic conditions such as diabetes, cardiovascular disease, and hypertension. These factors can generate more obstacles and more risk, and discontent mounts.

The Legal Template

Though there may be jurisdictional differences, once a duty to treat has been established, there are 3 additional elements to proving malpractice (**Fig. 3**).

The first element required to be proven is either negligence or the failure to act with ordinary care. This area usually involves expert witnesses and applicable literature. The battle is over whether the defendant acted unreasonably.

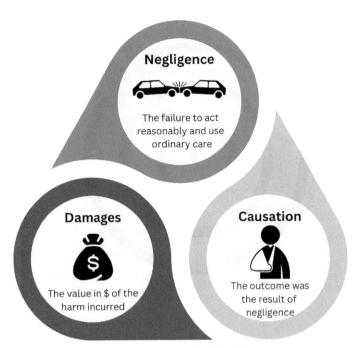

Fig. 3. Three core elements to proving a case of malpractice.

The second element is causation, which is basically whether the negligent acts resulted in a worse course or outcome than would have otherwise occurred with the rendering of appropriate care. The plaintiff's attorney will contend that but for the substandard and unreasonable care, the patient would have avoided the adverse outcome.

The third element is damages, or how the patient has been harmed by the negligent action of the health care provider. It is, of course, measured in money. The categories of damages can be both economic (eg, medical expenses and lost earnings) and noneconomic (eg, physical pain and mental anguish). These elements are interconnected in medical cases.

Making the Mark in the Emergency Department

There is no substitute for being proficient in judgment, documentation, and interpersonal dealings (**Fig. 4**). Obviously, education, training, and experience sharpen an already fine intellect; but having a *sixth sense* in clinical judgment is something that separates those who have a lot of legal problems, and those who do not. That sixth sense may be when something does not look quite right, or a test needs to be repeated, or a specialist needs to be consulted statim, Latin for immediately (STAT).

A recent review of diagnostic errors in the ED found a main cause to be inadequacies in the bedside diagnosis process, including medical reasoning, assessment, and decision-making.[7] The same study reported that malpractice claims pertaining to ED care had these factors 89% of the time, and uncommon case-specific variables that increased the cognitive challenge of care, such as atypical symptoms, were a predictor of mistakes in the ED.[7]

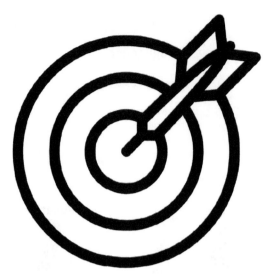

Fig. 4. Making the mark.

Documentation

Being adept at what to note in the records not only documents events, and reflects the level of judgment of the provider, but also protects. It is a journal of the main aspects of care and the central thoughts of the treating doctor. How important is this?

Consider that when a patient seeks an attorney to see if there is a case, the frequent routine is for the records to be obtained and reviewed by the law firm's nurse paralegal or an expert. The question "is there a case?" is often answered by what is reflected in the ED record. Inconsistencies and inaccuracies in the record raise questions about whether the record is correctly capturing what was said and what was done, and whether the communication that occurred in the ED was reflected in the record.[5] Lawyers know this.

Ghaith and colleagues have found that documentation issues frequently exist in lawsuits against emergency physicians, and the records are commonly the main source used by plaintiffs' lawyers for determining if the case is worth pursuing; poor records, including displaying inadequate, incorrect, or even information in conflict with other ED providers, can tip the scales toward a lawsuit being filed versus the lawyer telling the patient they do not have a viable case.[8]

Good bedside manner: there is no substitute

Finally, the variable of bedside manner by the treating physician is of, at least, equal importance to judgment and record keeping. I view it as pivotal. Manifesting characteristics like arrogance, insensitivity, unfriendliness, aloofness, uncaring, and sarcasm is a good way to trigger dissatisfaction in patients and their families. I have found it to be a significant factor in claims and lawsuits, and studies have long documented it.[3,9]

In a UK study by Vincent and colleagues entitled "Why do people sue doctors?," the original injury was compounded by the perception of poor communication by the treating doctors and insensitivity after the tragic event.[4] In this same study, patients and/or families were interviewed about their motivations for suing. Here are a couple of responses that apply across all medical specialties:

- "If I were to use a couple of words, they would be accountability and justice. To be more explicit, there seems to be an all-pervasive attitude that doctors are somehow above and beyond the normal restraints the rest of humanity have to abide by."[4]
- Another patient said, "the obstetrician said by way of an explanation 'it was just one of those things' (after death of a grandchild). That's not good enough – people need more than that... I feel no need for vengeance, witnessing the grief of my son and daughter-in-law hurt me so much and I felt desperate for them – I hope to get the answers they need."[4]

The numbers from the Vincent study are illuminating as to the feeling associated with pursuing a case: over 70% of respondents described themselves as having been severely affected by what had happened, feelings of anger were present in 90%, bitterness in 80%, betrayal in 55%, and humiliation in 40%.[4]

One example highlighting this is a physician I defended where an elderly man fell, later being diagnosed with a ruptured spleen. In the ED, before the diagnosis was made, the young physician made an unfortunate comment to the family which likely cemented him being included in the case as a defendant. He said, "isn't it about time for your dad to go into a nursing home?," something that the daughter recalled with some disdain when she testified in her deposition. She happened to be a lawyer.

This was a simple failure to "read the room," and the preferable default is that when a loved one is in dire straits, there is no need to lecture the family on their approach. Communication becomes more critical when there is distress.[4] Flippant commentary about weight, appearance, living situation, habits, or whether an elder family member can live on their own can leave the wrong kind of mark.

CASE STUDY 1
Facts

On June 21st, 2017, a Caucasian male individual, aged 53 years, presented to ER at 18:59 hours with chest pain, headache, nausea, shortness of breath, and acute burning constant radiating pain into the upper back for 1 hour prior to arrival. The pain began after the patient was cutting his grass. Triage at 19:00 hours by registered nurse (RN) noted the pain was diffuse. Pain was rated at 10 out of 10, and he was noted to be in severe distress.

At 19:21 hours, the ED physician noted a chief complaint of burning chest pain with abrupt onset that was associated with dizziness and radiated to his left shoulder and behind both ears. The physical examination was documented: "Apparent distress noted; alert, cooperative; moderate distress. Anxious and fidgety." An electrocardiogram (ECG) was taken at 19:03 hours and interpreted at 19:23 hours. The ECG showed "artifact, normal sinus rhythm; normal Axis; Q wave, R wave, and S wave (QRS) normal; S-T segment (ST) and or T waves normal." Additional documentation: Sat 100%, initially high blood pressure (BP) moderated with narcotics and anxiolytics, no ST changes.

Laboratories including complete blood count (CBC), chemistry, and troponin were normal. Computed tomography chest scan with contrast for chest pain reported "no dissection, no pericardial fluid, and no mediastinal lesion."

Doctor assessed the patient for costochondritis and lower sternal pain; xiphoid block acuity 3. Doctor administered bupivacaine into the periosteum of the lower sternum and xiphoid and documented that "pain improved after local anesthetic infiltration of the area of the pain with dramatic improvement. No change in chest pain

Commentary

Initial treatment with Aspirin 325mg dose
given; O2 by mask and cardiac monitoring
started- EKG done and compared with
2015- Cardiac Enz done and are
negative- no arrhythmias, no
pulmonary/respiratory symptoms, no
diaphoresis. However, with NTG paste
and iv Morphine Rx, Anxiolytic Rx several
minutes later caused a mod BP drop and
required a small fluid bolus and a 1-2
minute recumbent position- corrected
transient hypotension without recurrence.
Pain improved after local anesthetic
infiltration of the area of the pain with
dramatic improvement. No change in
chest pain with topical NTG although the
BP clearly responded secondarily
excluding cardiac source.

Reviewed;Nitropaste (nitroglycerin) 1
inch(es) has an Adverse Effect noted.

Reviewed;Ativan (lorazepam) 1 mg has
an Adverse Effect noted.

Fig. 5. Doctor's commentary.

with topical nitroglycerin (NTG) although the BP clearly responses secondarily excluding cardiac source" **(Fig. 5)**.

At 21:12 hours, Doctor notes "discharge: good condition; improved condition; stable condition; sent to home." Patient was discharged home at 22:00 hours.

The patient collapsed about an hour later, and the son observed seizure activity. He was transported by emergency medical services (EMS) to another hospital where a cardiologist documented that the patient arrived in ventricular fibrillation and was resuscitated with an ECG showing inferior ST elevation. He was emergently taken to the cardiac catheterization laboratory where it was found that he had a complete occlusion of the right and mid coronary artery. It was stented and the patient remained on the ventilator but unfortunately was found to have anoxic brain injury and was eventually pronounced dead.

Expert Feedback

1. ECG: ED doctor read the ECG as normal. He also commented that a previous ECG from 2015 was reviewed. Three ECGs were obtained on patient. The first 2 had a poor baseline. The third ECG had the best baseline of the 3, and it showed significant ST-segment depression in leads I and augmented vector left (aVL) as well as ST-segment depression of approximately 0.5 mm in leads V3 to V5, consistent with active ischemia. The previous ECG from 2015 is normal, clearly different than the ECG of June 21st, 2017.

2. Costochondritis: The diagnosis of costochondritis is not well supported by the documentation. It would be unusual for costochondritis pain at the xiphoid to radiate to the back, left shoulder, and to an area behind both ears. There is no documentation of increased pain with twisting or other torso maneuvers. There is no documentation of chest wall tenderness, redness, or swelling. Finally, the

documentation of a "dramatic" improvement with the xiphoid block is contradicted by the nursing documentation of pain only improving from an 8 out of 10 to a 5 out of 10.

3. Unstable angina: The history, though not diagnostic, is concerning for unstable angina. This 53 year old man was overweight, bordering on clinical obesity (body mass index 29.4), and is a smoker. He had exertional-onset pain with radiation to the left shoulder and ears. Doctor appeared to be considering cardiac ischemia based on the early administration of aspirin and nitrates; however, he did not follow through on this diagnosis and workup.

4. It would have been appropriate to apply a risk stratification tool for low-risk chest pain to this patient, the most common of which is the HEART score. Utilizing the HEART score, this patient would have scored at least 6 points (H = 2, E = 1, A = 1, R = 2, T = 0) and would, therefore, have warranted further in-patient or observation-unit workup before discharge.

5. Doctor suggested that the lack of pain improvement to the NTG paste excluded a cardiac source, but lack of response to NTG does not exclude a cardiac source; that is, NTG cannot be used as a diagnostic modality.[10,11]

6. It seems likely that if the decision had been made to admit the patient during his visit to ER, he would have been maintained on a monitor and could have been de-fibrillated immediately at the time of cardiac arrest.

Legal Considerations

- The opposing attorneys will attack on a "worst first" theory. A fatal cardiac condition should have been suspected as brewing, they will argue, such that there should have been a deep dive from the beginning to rule it out, and admitting the patient was the safest course.
- The record fails to convincingly detail why this was not a simmering cardiac condition and why it was, instead, a somewhat unusual musculoskeletal condition. This is key to the opposing attorney, and the argument will be that a budding catastrophic heart issue simply cannot be dismissed.
- Occam's razor will also be used by the opponent to underscore that the simplest explanation was a cardiac cause, and recognition of this should have been clear. To counter this argument, it is imperative to have better documentation in the chart that fully justifies the diagnosis of costochondritis and that thoroughly shows why a more hazardous cardiac condition was not what was happening.
- Tough questioning will follow:
  - Your records state that you have ruled out a cardiac condition as the cause of the decedent's symptoms. Do you agree you were wrong?
  - Do you agree that it would have been reasonable to have admitted this patient and consulted a specialist? What would the downside have been?
  - How often have you seen a patient with costochondritis?
  - How common is that condition? How often does it cause death?
  - Cardiac events are a common cause of death, correct? Would it have been safer for this patient for you to make sure this was not a cardiac event before sending him home?

CASE STUDY 2
Facts

On January 4th, 2017, a 43 year old man presented to the ED with several months of back pain. His decision to come to the hospital was prompted by an episode of incontinence that day including incontinence of both urine and stool in the ED (**Fig. 6**).

History of Present Illness:

01/04
04:02 This 43 years old White Male presents to ED via Walk-in with complaints of **sciatic pain**.

05:20 The patient presents with pain that is chronic, and decreased range of motion. The symptoms are located in the low back. The pain radiates to the left leg. The problem was sustained during a MVC, laminectomy last june. Onset: The symptoms/episode began/occurred gradually. Associated signs and symptoms: Pertinent positives: weakness, bowel incontinence, bladder incontinence. Severity of symptoms: At their worst the symptoms were moderate, in the emergency department the symptoms are unchanged. The patient has experienced similar episodes in the past, several times. The patient has not recently seen a physician, the patient's primary care provider is ███████ pt complains of increased pain to his back that radiates to his left leg, states he was incontinent of bowel and bladder. .

Fig. 6. Case study 2 report.

The nurse triaged him as level 3, and he was placed in the fast track where he saw a nurse practitioner (NP) who ordered a lumbar MRI. Due to "patient movement," the MRI was considered inconclusive by the radiologist.

The patient was in the ER for 5 hours and 27 minutes. He was eventually discharged with a prescription for Motrin and a diagnosis of lower back pain due to sciatica. He did not see the doctor, but the doctor signed off on the NP's discharge.

Less than 5 hours later the patient called EMS reporting weakness, saddle anesthesia, loss of bowel and bladder function, and complete lack of feeling in the extremities. He was taken to a different hospital where he was diagnosed with cauda equina syndrome (CES) and underwent surgery.

Legal Considerations

- Because the sequelae of CES can be so serious, they are also ripe for larger settlements.
- We obtained an independent expert review of this case and also requested that a literature search be done on CES. It was felt by the expert that the initial triage, which placed the patient on the track to see the NP, was probably incorrect. The complaint of incontinence upped the ante of a potential serious diagnosis with the expert hired by the defense opining that triage should have placed the patient in the main ED to see a physician.
- A rectal examination was done, which was good; but the result was a poor rectal tone. This finding, along with a report of prior incontinence, should have raised more concern. The NP pursued an MRI, which was a good idea.
- The MRI report emphasized the patient's movement and that opened up questions about how much reliance should be placed on it (**Fig. 7**).
- Summary: The patient comes to the ED with back pain, at least one episode of incontinence, has poor rectal tone, and the MRI is just not that helpful. Yet the patient is discharged, partly, because they observe him walk to go and smoke a cigarette outside.
- The opposing attorney will portray this as a simmering emergency, and that time is of the essence. Like a script, the main points will center around "what is the

IMPRESSION:
1. Patient motion severely limits the study.
2. Degenerative spondylosis with disc desiccation and facet joint hypertrophy mostly at L3-4, L4-5, and L5-S1. At L3-4 there is spinal canal stenosis. At L4-5 and L5-S1 there is probably some lateral recess stenosis but not well evaluated due to patient motion.

Fig. 7. MRI report impression.

downside admitting this patient to be seen by a specialist?" and "what is the danger to the patient if he has CES and you send him home?"

- Better notes, showing that CES or other significant conditions were considered and reasonably ruled out, are a necessity. It is, therefore, preferred to show in the record things like:
  - The incontinence was only one episode, and he has had it before;
  - The rectal tone was checked again and was stronger;
  - Saddle anesthesia was specifically evaluated, and the patient had appropriate feeling in the entire area, was able to urinate and have a bowel movement while in the ED, and was instructed about seeking immediate help if any further issues in these regards.
  - A specialist was consulted and agreed that based on the MRI, the patient could be discharged to follow up as an outpatient.
- The discharge instructions (**Fig. 8**) seem form-like, and, again, the failure to customize and note with precision what the patient was told is an area of vulnerability. Though new guidelines help cut down on note bloat,[12] meaty points on key areas are not frivolous verbiage. It is crucial that the record shows that clear and detailed instructions were covered with the patient, and that the plan is reasonable.

CASE STUDY 3: LIGHTNING ROUND
Chief Complaint: Left Eye Is Crusty and Hurts

- The complaint alleged that the ED physician failed to perform a thorough examination of a 60 year old patient's eye and misdiagnosed him with pink eye when he actually had acute angle closure glaucoma of the left eye. The patient ended up sustaining a 75% loss of vision.
- The ED physician took the position that the nurses did a visual acuity examination and told him it was normal. The examination is not noted, and his review of it is not noted.
- Opposing expert acknowledged the very atypical presentation of glaucoma with this patient. But he emphasized that "visual acuity is often considered to be a vital sign of the eye" and "it is the responsibility of the attending physician to review this data." He went on to emphasize in his report:
  - The standard of care requires performing a visual acuity examination and documented measurement of same. This opinion is supported by textbooks in emergency medicine and ophthalmology. I could find no literature that says that it is acceptable to not measure visual acuity with the presentation of no probleman ocular complaint."

Disposition:
01/05 Attestation: On the date of service, I reviewed the patient's history, exam findings, diagnostics and any
09:16 interventions or procedures in detail with the assigned midlevel provider and agreed with the care plan. Chart complete.

Diagnosis:
1. Back Pain w/ Sciatica

Disposition:
01/04
04:29 **01/04/2017 04:09 Discharged to Home/Self Care. Impression: Back Pain w/ Sciatica;. Condition is Stable. Discharge Instructions: BACK PAIN W/ SCIATICA. Prescriptions for Ibuprofen 800 mg Oral Tablet - take 1 tablet by ORAL route every 8 hours As needed; 30 tabletFollow up: Private Physician; When: 2 - 3 days; Reason: Worsening of conditions, Continuance of care. Problem is new. Symptoms are**

Fig. 8. Discharge instructions.

- Bottom line: Either the visual acuity examination was done, and reviewed, and no documentation happened, or it was not done. The recurring problem is the failure to note what has been done. If it was done and documented, there is no case. The failure to record it raises questions of whether it happened, and when a serious injury follows, such as a large loss of vision in one eye, a plaintiff's attorney will see the opening for a case by the lack of evidence of a basic examination being done.[8]

CASE STUDY 4: CHIEF COMPLAINT: A 5 YEAR OLD PRESENTS WITH SYMPTOMS OF CORONAVIRUS DISEASE 2019 OR FLU

- The complaint alleged that the doctor "slapped the patient on the buttocks, after completing examination and discussing the case with the patient's parents, resulting in the patient crying at the unprofessional action."
- The ED physician responded:
  - After my initial evaluation, I ordered COVID, flu, and unstable angina (UA) testing, which all came back negative. I concluded that she was suffering from a generic viral syndrome with the possibility of a false-negative COVID study given early presentation. I discussed the findings of my physical examination, work-up, and treatment plan with the patient's parents and they understood the discharge instructions and plan. Next is when I patted the patient on her bottom and she was startled.
  - After the patient cried, I apologized to the patient and her parents. Her father did not seem to react but her mother was upset and said that while she appreciated what I did as her physician, I should not have touched her daughter's 'private area.' She asked to speak with a supervisor."
- Bottom line: This is a judgment issue. Years ago, this would probably have not been viewed as a big deal by very many parents. Times are different now, and more care must be taken. I recommend being very discreet in what is said and what is done when it comes to casual conversation or conduct in the ED. In some regards, boundaries are more present than ever, and people have hair-triggers when it comes to complaining about a boundary violation.
  - A better option than patting the little girl on the bottom to celebrate that she does not have the flu or coronavirus disease 2019? How about saying "give your folks a high-5 at these good test results"?

CASE STUDY 5
Facts

A girl was born April 5th, 2011, 6 weeks premature. Soon after delivery, she had difficulty breathing, and she was transferred to a children's hospital and placed under an oxygen hood. She also had thrombocytopenia, hyperbilirubinemia, and metabolic acidosis, which were treated.

She had an intravenous (IV) line placed in her left foot for peritoneal nutrition. On April 14, she received a hepatitis B shot on her left thigh. She was discharged home.

On Saturday, April 20, around midnight, the parents brought her, now 15 days old, to an ER near their home. They were concerned about a fever that had started a few hours before, and they complained of redness and swelling at the IV sight and at the location of the shot on the thigh.

The ED doctor noted slight induration at the thigh, which he attributed to the shot. He noted redness at the sight of the IV. He diagnosed phlebitis. He prescribed oral antibiotics (amoxicillin) and told the parents to see the pediatrician (they already had an appointment in 2 days). The child was not admitted, no laboratories were done, and no consultations were obtained.

On the 22nd, they went to the pediatrician's office. There was no temperature, but the redness and swelling had spread through the entire leg. The pediatrician sent them to the children's hospital. There she was diagnosed with cellulitis, phlebitis, thrombophlebitis, osteomyelitis, and a septic left hip. She had surgery and experienced a limb length deformity.

Expert Feedback

The plaintiff expert stated after reviewing the records "pretty much every recommendation you read is that a kid under 90 days (especially a kid under 30 days), you have to assume it is a severe infection and have to work her up and admit her." Blood work should have been done, and the baby should have either been admitted or sent back to the children's hospital.

The expert was also dissatisfied with the discharge instructions. She felt that saying "go to the PCP in 2 to 3 days" is not sufficient. She felt that the prescription of amoxicillin was inappropriate as this should not be done in a newborn without blood cultures.

Legal Considerations

- A barrage of questions would be lodged by the child's attorney to the ED doctor:
  ○ What would have been the downside to obtaining blood work?
  ○ Why not assume it was potentially a serious infection and try to rule that out?
  ○ What would be the risk to admitting the baby and consulting a specialist? What was the risk of not doing so?
  ○ Why not instruct the parents to take the child to the pediatrician when the office is opened in a few hours rather than merely keeping a pre-existing appointment in 2 days?
- In my view, a baby with a fever is in a different category as far as concern and action needed. Members of a jury will likely expect *extra* effort to make sure that serious conditions are ruled out.
- Worth noting is the skimpy nature of the discharge instructions (**Fig. 9**) on a midnight run to the ER by a family regarding a 15 day old premature baby with a fever and swollen leg. Diagnosis: the generic "cellulitis." Does this family understand this? Hard to say since there is nothing else noted about a discussion with them. A cryptic "call referral doc in 2 to 3 days for re-evaluation" is the instruction, and what happens if that call is not returned for a day or two?
- Patients and families often do not understand the care that took place or the instructions given upon discharge from the ED.[13] This is an area where it seems to me that corners are often cut, and it is a task that appears to be frequently

Care provided by Dr. ███████████ MD with the diagnosis of .

Thanks again for using ████████████████ for your treatment today. The discharge instructions for today's visit are outlined below.

Cellulitis
Amoxicillin 250 mg / 5 cc
Call referral doc in 2-3 days for re-evaluation

Special Notes:

Fig. 9. Discharge instructions.

lateraled to the facility staff. Yet, it is a crucial part of the record and less than stellar discharge instructions can fuel a lawsuit.

SUMMARY

There is no way to guarantee a medical career that is free of complaints, claims, or lawsuits. Too many variables are at play, and ultimately there is no way to stop someone from acting on their dissatisfaction; however, there are measures that can minimize the risk of claims being made.

Clinicians can exercise great judgment, create good records, and display solid interpersonal skills with others. Success in these areas can dramatically lessen adverse events and associated claims, which saves you from risk and some unpleasant rides. Good luck!

CLINICS CARE POINTS

- Clinic care points in these regards would include working through indicated diagnosis and care algorithms, coordinating and integrating care, noting the important information and results in the chart, and showing respect and empathy for the patient and family.
- Properly purusing continuity and transition of care, whether the patient is being admitted or being discharged to follow up, is pivotal as well.

DISCLOSURE

The author has nothing to disclose concerning financial interests. Artificial intelligence was a help in creating some of the original images in this article.

REFERENCES

1. King G, Charles proteus steinmetz, the wizard of schenectady. Smithsonian.com, Available at: https://www.smithsonianmag.com/history/charles-proteus-steinmetz-the-wizard-of-schenectady-51912022/, (Accessed October 1, 2023), 2011.
2. Jena AB, Seabury S, Lakdawalla D, et al. Malpractice risk according to physician specialty. N Engl J Med 2011;365(7):629–36.
3. Hickson GB. Patient complaints and malpractice risk. JAMA 2002;287(22):2951.
4. Vincent C, Phillips A, Young M. Why do people sue doctors? a study of patients and relatives taking legal action. Lancet 1994;343(8913):1609–13.
5. Yu KT, Green RA. Critical aspects of emergency department documentation and communication. Emerg Med Clin 2009;27(4):641–54.
6. Wong K, Parikh PD, Miller K, et al. Emergency department and urgent care medical malpractice claims 2001–15. West J Emerg Med 2021;22(2).
7. Newman-Toker DE, Peterson SM, Badihian S, et al. Diagnostic Errors in the Emergency Department: A Systematic Review [Internet]. Rockville (MD): Agency for Healthcare Research and Quality (US); 2022. (Comparative Effectiveness Review, No. 258.) Available at: https://www.ncbi.nlm.nih.gov/books/NBK588118/. doi: 10.23970/AHRQEPCCER258.
8. Ghaith S, Moore G, Colbenson K, et al. Charting practices to protect against malpractice: case reviews and learning points. West J Emerg Med 2022;23(3):412–7.
9. Sloan FA, Mergenhagen PM, Burfield WB, et al. Medical malpractice experience of physicians. Predictable or haphazard? JAMA 1989;262(23):3291–7.

10. Gulati M, Levy PD, Mukherjee D, et al. 2021 AHA/ACC/ASE/CHEST/SAEM/SCCT/ SCMR Guideline for the Evaluation and Diagnosis of Chest Pain: A Report of the American College of Cardiology/American Heart Association Joint Committee on Clinical Practice Guidelines. Circulation 2021;144(22):e368–454 [published correction appears in Circulation. 2021 Nov 30;144(22):e455] [published correction appears in Circulation. 2023 Dec 12;148(24):e281].
11. Diercks DB, Boghos E, Guzman H, et al. Changes in the numeric descriptive scale for pain after sublingual nitroglycerin do not predict cardiac etiology of chest pain. Ann Emerg Med 2005;45(6):581–5.
12. Marshall K, Strony RS, Hohmuth B, et al. New coding guidelines reduce emergency department note bloat but more work is needed. Ann Emerg Med 2023;82(6):713–7.
13. Engel KG. Patient comprehension of emergency department care and instructions: are patients aware of what they don't understand? Acad Emerg Med 2006;13(5Supplement 1):S101.

Moving?

Make sure your subscription moves with you!

To notify us of your new address, find your **Clinics Account Number** (located on your mailing label above your name), and contact customer service at:

Email: journalscustomerservice-usa@elsevier.com

800-654-2452 (subscribers in the U.S. & Canada)
314-447-8871 (subscribers outside of the U.S. & Canada)

Fax number: 314-447-8029

Elsevier Health Sciences Division
Subscription Customer Service
3251 Riverport Lane
Maryland Heights, MO 63043

*To ensure uninterrupted delivery of your subscription, please notify us at least 4 weeks in advance of move.

.